To the team &
working forum,

Stay Positive
&
be awesome

Heath
☺

Breaking the Mirror

by

Heather Wright

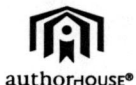
authorHOUSE®

AuthorHouse™
1663 Liberty Drive, Suite 200
Bloomington, IN 47403
www.authorhouse.com
Phone: 1-800-839-8640

© 2007 Heather Wright. All rights reserved.

No part of this book may be reproduced, stored in a retrieval system, or transmitted by any means without the written permission of the author.

First published by AuthorHouse 10/24/2007

ISBN: 978-1-4259-6802-1 (sc)

Printed in the United States of America
Bloomington, Indiana

This book is printed on acid-free paper.

"All men dream: but not equally. Those who dream by night in the dusty recesses of their minds wake in the day to find that it was vanity: but the dreamers of the day are dangerous men, for they may act their dreams with open eyes, to make it possible."

T.E. Lawrence,
The Seven Pillars of Wisdom.

Breaking the Mirror

By
Heather Wright of Advance Performance

Kagami Biraki or *Breaking The Mirror* is a traditional Japanese ceremony held at the beginning of each year for the students of Aikido at the Yoshinkan Dojo (training hall) – where the Tokyo Riot Police Train in the Martial Art of Aikido (the way of Harmony).

The mirror, we are told, contains the old image: we look on it with old eyes and memories of who we believe ourselves to be and yet every cell in our body is different from the cells we had six months ago. We are new every moment and have the possibility of breaking the old confines and becoming a new person.

A new version of ourselves.

Breaking the Mirror

The miracle question is this ...

> If you woke up tomorrow and your life was exactly how you want it to be, what would it look like?

If you were to re-invent yourself right now I have no doubt that you would choose to lose the bad habits and keep the good, to lose the things about you that you do not like and to encourage the parts that you love, in fact to enhance them so that they become a major part of your persona.

You may even choose to adopt some new habits. You would become a better person, and our choice as to what that better person was like, would be ours and ours alone.

I have, for quite a few years now, devoted myself to helping others achieve their goals and dreams; helping them to become the people that they believe they can be. During this period of my life I have noticed, time and again, that some people seize upon this philosophy of living (for that is what it is) and change their lives for ever, never looking back, but they are fewer than I would ever have thought.

Does this tell us that success is only available to a select few? **Is God selective about our ability to be successful** (in whatever way we choose to define success)?

In my opinion, this cannot be the case. But, as with many of our gifts, we each have talents that come easily and many more that come less so, which need working on, sometimes on a daily basis.

It is my belief that we can achieve pretty much all that we wish to. Our only true limitation is time, and because none of us have the wonderful lifespan of Methuselah we must prioritise, but more about that later.

Let us compare our mental work out with a physical one. We all know how important it is to keep healthy and because jobs and daily routines, no longer involve as much physical effort as they once did, we have to make extra time for it.

Only a small percentage of people actually spend time achieving any level of fitness above the norm. Those who do often arrange to meet a friend to attend a particular class that they like or they get into a routine of attending a class at a set time. Those with more disposable income may pay a personal trainer to take them through the necessary work out.

This book is your personal trainer; it should not be put on a shelf somewhere and kept clean for fear of creasing the spine. It should be left somewhere to remind you everyday what area you are developing that day. You may wish to leave it in the bathroom; you may wish to have it in your car, in your gym bag or on your coffee table. I now keep books with me everywhere I go; let's not waste any of the wonderful time we have been so generously given.

This book is designed to give a little something to think about and work on every couple of days.

Only three sessions per week.

I once read a Bible Study book by Charles Swindoll which was three sessions a week; it is the only bible study book I have completed, I kept it going for the whole year, I rarely got behind and if I did, I could catch up easily. It was manageable and if I was feeling good, instead of reading ahead I would read the same section two days running.

This is what I would recommend you to do with this book. Each subsection has a short amount of text to read and then some questions for you to think about and make a note of. Then I would suggest that you continue to think about the questions and your answers for the following day or two and if necessary come back to it a couple of times.

Write the question down and place it somewhere to remind you. I do not claim to be perfect or know more than anyone else, I only wish to stimulate your thoughts, to encourage you to question the status quo as others have done for me.

If you disagree with what I have put that's great - at least I have encouraged you to think about it.

> **Get a highlighter and a pen or pencil and write in this book, doodle, highlight, personalise it, make it your journal of personal development.**

You may have heard some of it before, that's great, and I don't intend to be a revolutionary. Most of the material in this book is in the public domain, and so it should be, personal development belongs to anyone who wants it and seeks it out.

Our job as speakers, authors, teachers, mothers, fathers, children and friends is to share it generously. After all, the impact we make on others is the only thing that lives on after we have gone.

Let's not fool ourselves – **the impact can be either positive or negative.** In order for us to move forward it must surely be our goal for that impact to be positive.

Over 9 years ago two colleagues (Michael Finnigan and Andrew O'Donoghue) and I formed a company to pursue our vision, the company is Advance Performance.

Our Vision is this:

A better world for this and future generations

Heather Wright

What's yours?

1

The Air Hostess School of Thinking

When anyone travels by plane nowadays, after we have se
into our seats and the aircraft is positioned in the que
take off, the air hostess or a video of an air hostess
through the safety procedures. Personally I would
contemplate crashing before we have even left
but I understand the need.

At some point during this speech he or she
along the lines of "if you have a small c
make sure you fit your own mask first h
needs of your child".

Heather Wright

It may seem a pretty selfish thing to do, to help yourself first; it's a tough decision for a parent.

But surely we are of no use to the child if, half way through helping them, we are asphyxiated and cannot finish the job.

If we put our own mask on first we can follow the job through.

The same is true in other walks of life, before we can help anyone else we must surely get ourselves, at least partially sorted out first. Who would want to listen to our advice on marriage if we are currently handling our relationships badly?

"m not suggesting we have to be perfect before we attempt to elp others, that is a quite a journey and if anyone completes efore they die please would you write to me and let me w how they achieved it. But we must at least be on the path.

people may say why should we change at all?

fore we go any further write down on the next page the t important things in your life.

Breaking the Mirror

The 5 most important things in my life are …

1. My wife Deborah

2. Our family

3. Our health.

4. Fulfilment in everything we do!

5. Financially secure for us and anyone who needs our help

Take a moment now to reflect on those five things.

Heather Wright

The journey of our own development is about the important things; not about keeping the boss happy (although this can be good too) nor is it about many of the other things we worry about on a daily basis.

It is about the things that are important. Is there an area for improvement in your life that, will add to your quality of life? Will make you happier and help with those things that are important to you?

Write down the five words that describe you at your best.

1. Contented

2. Grateful.

3. Fit

4. In practice ~~& it~~

5. Loving

Breaking the Mirror

How often do you achieve them?

65% % of the time

How often would you like to achieve them?

100% % of the time

If the first number is smaller than the second one then we can start working on it straight away.

Write down some of the times you achieve those five best behaviours.

> **Action ...**
>
> Now spend some time over the next day or so, becoming aware of the times when you deviate from your best behaviours and why.

2

Zing and Zap

✟

Are we talking about two aliens from a cartoon strip? No, Zing stands for salt or flavour and Zap is light. Both salt and light are essential for sustaining life. Salt was once as valuable a commodity as gold, and in the first millennium traders would trade it, pound for pound. So, what does salt do? It preserves food and it adds flavour.

In recent times so much salt is put into our food in order to preserve it and make it tasty that we are told we have to stop adding it as it hardens our arteries and is therefore bad for our hearts.

Flavour (Zing) is essential, but we cut it out. When we are small children life is exciting, everything is exciting even a car trip from the house to the shops is exciting. My youngest son finds everyday amazing; he runs round sucking the life out of life itself, enjoying every moment, the worst thing you can say to him is "its bed time". You can see the look in his eyes that says "but I haven't finished with today yet – how can it be over?" From the moment he wakes up he is switched on totally, he wouldn't ever dream of rolling over in bed saying "Oh no, not another day – just five more minutes sleep, please".

At some point in our lives we have all been like that. But we have changed, now we turn into bed worshippers, we fall unceremoniously out of our pit onto the floor turn and kiss the warm bed saying "I'll be back soon, don't miss me too much". Then we set that all important goal – to return to bed as soon as we can manage it.

What happened? Where did the flavour go? When did we start cutting it out? My theory is that during our teenage years, we believe it is cool to be bored with everything and that to be excited is childish, so we learn to cut out the flavour. What a shame.

Did you know that the average child laughs 400 times a day and the average adult laughs 15 times a day?

Light (Zap) is also essential but when we have been in the dark for a while and someone switches on the light it hurts our eyes, so we hide under the duvet. Blaming the light for the pain.

We are the same with enthusiasm and excitement. When was the last time you met someone who really enjoyed their job and showed it? Someone who gets enthusiastic about events coming up? We laugh at them and call them naïve. Maybe it's us that have it wrong.

Mark Twain once said "A cat that sits on a hot stove will never sit on a hot stove ever again. But then it won't sit on a cold one either". The point I believe he was trying to make is that we, like the cat, experience pain either physical or psychological and blame the wrong thing for it.

We choose to believe that when someone is full of energy, enthusiasm or excitement, they are at fault. Maybe they have lost the plot, don't understand how difficult life is or aren't very 'realistic'.

What a pity, who are we trying to impress? This isn't a rehearsal; this life is the real McCoy, its one chance. Let's start enjoying it a little bit more. Let's turn the light up a bit and add more flavour.

Write down a few things that you really enjoy doing and look forward to doing with eager anticipation.

> **Action ...**
>
> Plan to do more things you enjoy more often, but also try to learn to enjoy more things, laugh at more jokes no matter how corny. It may feel odd at first; try not to cap your enjoyment. Watch other people for the next couple of days and notice their enjoyment levels and in particular the times they prevent themselves from becoming happier.

3
Yes People

✟

When I was expecting my first child, my husband and I joined an NCT (National Childbirth Trust) Group, so that we would know a little more about what was going on.

There were four couples in the class and as we got nearer to the births the four women stopped working and we met together for lunch once a week.

We gradually got fatter and fatter; I expect that not all of it was due to being pregnant! After we had given birth we met a few more times but gradually we lost touch.

Seven years later I met one of them when we were out for a drink one night, when she saw me she squealed with delight, gave me a huge hug abandoned her friends for at least half an hour to come over for a catch up chat. I saw quite a bit of her over the next year or so and found out that she and her husband had split up and she had had many other trials and tribulations in her life. Something she said to me one day really stuck with me.

The night before her daughter had a friend round for the night and the friend had been complaining about her mum and dad and had said to my friend's daughter "It's OK for you, you have a YES mum!"

My friend did not have plenty of money, she was a single parent struggling to make ends meet, have some social life and fit in time for working without being away from her daughter. She was not able to give her daughter everything she would have liked to but she was still a 'YES' mum. She said to me that she would start with the assumption that the answer was going to be yes and work out a way to make it happen.

Charles Swindoll writes in one of his books about having a 'YES' face. We all know people who have a 'NO' face. They start with the assumption that the answer is no and then work out how to justify it and it thus becomes part of their features. Maybe we should all learn to say 'YES' more often and smile more often. It will come from a

'YES' attitude. This doesn't apply to those of you who say 'YES' all the time and then don't have time for yourselves or your families.

**Are you a 'YES' person?
Or a 'YES BUT' person?
Or are you a 'NO' person?**

In some recent research done with teachers their entire conversations inside the class rooms were monitored. Even those teachers who perceived that they were positive during a pre-research interview scored less than 5% of positive comments.

The researcher told me that she had pretty wide boundaries, the phrase "Sit down" was deemed to be negative, but the phrase "Sit down please" was positive. So I ask again, are you a 'YES' person? Listen to your conversations over the next day or two and give your self a mark out of ten below.

Current perception of self   /10

Perception after a few days   /10

Breaking the Mirror

Write down here your perceptions of others you think are 'YES' people and 'NO' people try and find three of each.

'YES' people

'NO' people

What distinguishes between the two groups of people?

4
Best Behaviour

✠

When we run seminars at Advance, we often ask the people present what they are like at their best, just as I asked you to write down five words that describe you at your best during the first session of this book.

Words such as 'happy', 'confident', 'enthusiastic', 'effective' and 'calm' are often on the list. Occasionally words such as 'awesome', 'dynamic', 'buzzing' and 'unstoppable' are used. There are a variety of best behaviours and I think we would all agree that the best behaviour we require is the most appropriate behaviour for that particular time.

Breaking the Mirror

In order for a person to win an event such as the Tour De France they are not required to start the race one day and pedal like mad for three weeks and not stop until it is finished.

Each participant is required to use different tactics on different days. Some days they will have a short fast ride, sometimes it will be a longer flat ride (often in excess of 120 miles) and some days they ride as a team with all 9 members together taking it in turns to ride at the front and feel the wind resistance; some days are mountain stages when the climbers come into their own, and of course, after the climbs there are descents which are a speciality for some riders; in addition they have two well earned rest days as it is just as important to rest in the correct way.

When we look at best behaviour we are asking for the most effective behaviour at any one time.

So, how did you describe yourself at your best during the first few pages?

Would you like to change those words?

Write them again (or the words you would like to use now) on the next page.

1.

2.

3.

4.

5.

Are those words good enough? Are we aiming high enough? I am often told that there is nothing wrong with the word 'happy' and I have to agree that it is certainly better that 'misery' but its not much to aim for. Is there something better?

I have met a few depressives on my travels and those with mood swings tell me that once they start to get happy or even ecstatic they begin to tell themselves it won't last and become frightened. It is better not to aim so high, they tell me, than to feel the fear of it not lasting.

A gentleman recently told me that his life was all about survival, nothing more, because he was working class and that was all he could hope for. It seems to me that these people suffer from the same faulty reasoning.

> 'Whatever you do, don't aim too high then you can't be disappointed!!'

My argument is that we should aim high and learn to handle disappointment in an inspiring way, in a way that says "that was fantastic, how can I, get more?", rather than being obsessed about the fact that we aren't up there any more.

If you could have any sort of behaviours which would you like? If you really were raising the game what would you aim for?

No matter what your job is, or whether you are at home or on holiday.

Being at your best isn't just reserved for great sportspeople and actors who achieve large amounts of "feel good factor" from short term goals.

> Action ...
>
> Spend some time concentrating on best behaviour today; from time to time remind yourself what you are aiming for.

Consider ...

"What would the best parent do in these circumstances?"

"What would the best cleaner do right now?"

"How would the best friend answer this question?"

No matter what you are doing over the next couple of days consider what 'BEST' really is

5

Behaviour – Homer Syndrome

☦

I'm not a big Homer Simpson fan but my son is. I have noticed how often he speaks like Homer now and it drives me to distraction. Especially the expression "doh". Ever wondered what Homer means by it? I think he means "Why did I do that … again?" with the implication "I'm always doing that!"

Hands up anyone who has never in their life wondered why it seems to be so easy to do and say the stupid things in life over and over and how hard it is to repeat those moments of pure genius. If we could find that formula we'd be millionaires.

When I was growing up I just accepted that it was the job of everyone around me to point out what I was doing wrong. It just seemed to me that it was a constant. In other words there was very little I did right and a great deal of "Homer Simpson" moments. So much so, that in many areas of my life I had a pretty low opinion of my abilities. Luckily it didn't cover every area. My ability to act the fool scored very highly. My ability to win boyfriends (and then get bored with them very quickly) scored highly. These two abilities aren't subjects that registered very highly on my teachers list of 'How to get somewhere in life', but I guess it just depends on what you are focussing on.

So, having seen a wonderful film called, 'Freaky Friday' with Jodie Foster, I decided the only way to change was to swap places with someone else. Every morning I'd wake up and still be me though. Quite a disappointment!

I wonder how many children spend their lives wanting to be someone else. I'd like to think that as adults we have learned to appreciate our skills and better qualities. Focussing on what makes us unique and special rather than on what lets us down. But time and time again I come across people who are consistently pointing out to themselves or others their areas of weakness and their faults.

OK let's do an exercise.

Give yourself one minute to write down 5 things that make you outstanding:

1.

2.

3.

4.

5.

How did you do? Did you find it easy or hard?

Was it the time pressure? Or was it just that we are no good at thinking of ourselves as outstanding?

What about writing five qualities that make you 'alright'?

Is that easier?

Would you prefer five things you would like to change about yourself?

From now on I would like you to start noticing the things you do right and start writing them down.

Find in yourself qualities that make you the potential genius you are.

It may not be an academic skill such as Maths or English but they are only a couple of the many ways to be intelligent.

Include your ability to talk, or your ability to understand how people feel. What about your ability to love unconditionally? Or organise yourself to maximise efficiency?

Notice your awesome moments instead of the 'doh' ones.

Breaking the Mirror

Over the next couple of days, write down below …

Some of the things you have done that made you happy

Made someone else happy (or laugh – in a good way!)

Made you proud:

Made you glad to be you:

Heather Wright

Quick Recall Session

- Stop trying to change the world and start by sorting yourself out
- Focus on being unstoppable, buzzing, enthusiastic and whatever else you wrote down as your best behaviours
- Remember to enjoy life again – add some flavour
- Turn your dimmer switch up – for your own sake
- Be a 'YES' person – plan to talk about what can be done more often instead of what can't be done
- Smile more
- Aim for 100% best behaviour not mediocrity
- Concentrate on the things that make you special not on the things that don't
- Be yourself – be the best version of you that you can be

> "To accept one's past – one's history –
> Is not the same thing as drowning in it;
> It is learning how to use it."
>
> James Baldwin, Writer

Heather Wright

6

Isn't Life Exciting?!

✝

I have been reading today about a chap called John Goddard. Now, if you are from the USA you may have heard of him, if you aren't from America you may not.

When he was 15 John Goddard wrote a list of things he wanted to do. On this list were 127 things like, climb the highest mountain, travel the length of the Nile, read an entire encyclopaedia, ride on an elephant, learn to play Au Clair du Lune on the piano and many more. Since that time he has completed 109 of them. He was the first man to explore the whole length of the Nile – two other men went with him. He also contracted a tape worm he called

Rodney (they paddled a kayak each to complete it). He has retraced Marco Polo's route through all of the Middle East, Asia and China. He has lived with 260 different tribal groups; he has climbed Ararat, Kilimanjaro and Fuji. He has flown 47 different types of plane and been to 120 countries and what's more he is married with five children.

In order to do these things, he has nearly died many times, he was charged by hippos, crocodiles, a furious warthog and bloodsucking leeches (although I don't think they charge very often) in the Congo. He has survived plan crashes, earthquakes; three times he has been trapped in quick sand and almost drowned twice. He is now 74 and still has things to do including visit the moon. Hang in there John! I believe Richard Branson is selling tickets!!

This may not be your cup of tea, some of them don't appeal to me either, and you don't have to have a love of the dangerous to feel fulfilled, but it is surely necessary to feel that you are doing something with your life.   It takes all sorts to make up this world; different people with a wide variety of desires and passions.

But, what burning ambition do you have? What would you like to be able to say at your next dinner party ... "I am going to ... next week" or "oh yes, I've done that". Nowadays most things are possible, I bought my husband a flying lesson in a Tigermoth for Christmas and a day white water rafting (I have his insurance fully paid up). We've swum with dolphins and been to Lapland to meet Father Christmas, done free fall parachuting as well as jumping from high bridges into rivers. They aren't massive things but each thing was an experience never to be missed.

Life is about experiences, some are born out of necessity and we are forced into them, maybe we could choose a few extra ones to add flavour and spice. Let's not just exist, let's live a little. Oh stuff it, let's live a lot!

What have you always wanted to do? Go on start planning today.

Why not dream for a moment, write down ten things over the next couple of pages, that you would like to do at some time. Our restrictions are often not about money but about putting the effort in. I once met a lady who did set herself a different task each year – it had started when she was forty and realised she couldn't even drive, so she said to herself within the year I will learn to drive. When that year was over she was so pleased with herself, she set herself another task, maybe it was as simple as signing on for a Chinese Cookery course, it doesn't matter, its about purpose and experience.

So, back to the list:

1.

2.

3.

4.

5.

6.

7.

8.

9.

10.

If you haven't managed ten yet think about it over the next couple of days and ask yourself the following question ...

Breaking the Mirror

"What would I dare to attempt if I knew, without a doubt, I couldn't fail?

7

Motivation and Hope

✞

I am often asked to speak to groups of people on the subject of motivation. The client tells everyone there's a motivational speaker coming, half of the audience dread it and the other half look forward to someone larger than life, with a huge personality to leap onto the stage and shout so called 'motivational phrases' at them such as "you gotta look in the mirror and say 'I love me'."

Of course when I turn up it can often be a bit of a shock. I am, of course, one of those loud people, sorry, I can't help it I just get very excited about my subject. But I think it is important to make it clear that motivation comes from within you and not from me. I can stand on the stage and make you laugh and get you excited and it could all wear off by the morning, or if not, within a week.

True motivation, in my opinion, comes from our hope in our future and therefore the reverse is often true. Let me give you an example to see if I can clarify this point.

Imagine that you are sitting reading this book, your stomach is full, you are warm enough, you have clothes on your back that look pretty good, your mortgage is paid and your family is safe – BUT you know that next week something disastrous is going to happen and all of this will change; your family will abandon you, you will be hungry, your house will be taken away and there is nothing you can do about it. No matter how things are today, there will inevitably be stress and worry about next week; it may even become completely debilitative.

OK lets reverse that idea imagine that today you have nothing, you are sleeping on a friends sofa or on a park bench, you are hungry, you have been wearing the same old clothes for weeks, maybe months, but you know that next week all this will change, you will then have a home, food, a job, clothes etc. Today you will feel pretty good.

I believe that it is our hope in our future that inspires us. We suffer most from avoidant behaviour when we firmly believe that there is nothing we can do or that whatever we do will not be good enough.

In order to motivate people (including ourselves) we have to give each individual a picture of personal success. In order to do that we must first find out what they (we) want. Most of us give up at something when we realise that we are never going to get any better. We must believe that there is a future of constant improvement.

It is our hope in our future that motivates us and many of us aren't motivated by how effective we are at work. It is about being a better parent, partner, friend or sportsperson.

A couple of sessions ago I asked you to write down what the most important things in your life were. Go back and have a quick look at what you wrote.

Now I would like you to think about success. What is your definition of success? Write it below …

It can be a hard one, so why not just write down lots of bits of ideas and then over the next couple of days, think about it. Consider the people you think are most successful, I would be surprised if you come up with a list of only the rich and famous.

Look at the people around you as well as those you haven't met but have heard of. What makes them successful? What makes us happy?

8

Dare to Achieve

☦

When we are children we dream of what we can be when we are older. So far my children have wanted to be Batman, a toy factory owner who gives all the toys away free, a scientist and a palaeontologist. As we grow up we gradually learn to curb our dreams to be more realistic. How sad.

I have a friend who always wanted to be a Doctor instead he became a VAT inspector. When I asked him if he failed the exams he said that he never took them because he wasn't clever enough. I wonder how many years one would have to study to pass the exams eventually.

It's a bit like driving tests; people take them two, three or even four or five times in order to pass them. I hardly ever hear of people who say that driving is something they could never possibly pick up.

Learning languages is a similar thing, how many of us left school believing that we are "no good at languages" and yet if we were lost in any foreign country for a couple of months, maybe even a year or two we would learn the language. The only people I have ever known who have not succeeded were those who stubbornly refused to try or spent all their time with people who spoke English. One lady in the hotel industry told me that she had a member of her staff who had lived in England for many years and still could not speak the language but had managed to pick up Spanish because her boyfriend was Spanish – obviously desire is important.

Do you remember a television programme where Cilla Black used to show up on people's door steps and give a family member a seemingly impossible task to learn during the next week? If they successfully completed the task in front of a studio audience the following week they would get to choose many wonderful prizes from new cars, amazing holidays as well as gifts for the children. I watched, mesmerised, as a gentleman managed to place a tumbler over five dice and with a flick of the wrist remove the tumbler to reveal all five dice stacked neatly on top of one another, another lady had to memorise 50 or more pictures of golf courses and at random had to correctly identify each one. It's amazing what we can do if we really want to.

Recently there has been a programme on called 'Faking It' – an ordinary individual is given four weeks to learn how to do a job which is totally different from their own. They are given expert tuition, acting lessons and even a new hair style and image. They have successfully turned a sheep shearer into a professional hairdresser, a burger cook into a top chef, a painter and decorator into an artist, a go-go dancer into a horse rider, a ballet dancer into a wrestler and a Naval Officer into a drag queen. There is no big prize at the end except short lived television fame and feel good factor. Each 'victim' has to successfully enter either a competition or be judged by experts by being put alongside three or four others who are full time professionals to see if they are spotted. Once again, it is amazing what we can do if we really want to.

What is it you would like to do but think you can't? How much do you really want to do it? Are you making assumptions that are holding you back? Recently in a newspaper, I read an article about a man who suddenly decided to give up his job to study to become an accountant – he had to sell his house to pay for the tuition and study for three or more years, but he was prepared to do it, to achieve his goal. I read a similar article about a mechanic who decided to become a doctor, he had to start by getting the right 'O' levels and then on to 'A' levels before even attempting University.

What would you be prepared to put up with, if it meant you would achieve your goal?

9

Survival

✜

Helen Keller is quoted as saying "Life is either a daring adventure or nothing." – Of course this quote will mean nothing to you unless you know something of her background – she was deaf, blind, mute and born in the 19th Century when people with disabilities were treated as freaks and often put into institutions. A way of teaching her was devised and after much difficulty she became a campaigner, travelling around the world 'speaking' about her life and the challenges faced by those with disabilities like hers. She raised a lot of money for the blind and also became a political activist.

Heather Wright

Considering that she was a blind, deaf, mute, woman living in the 19th Century she was pretty amazing.

I was speaking at a company recently when a rather unhappy looking chap spent a great deal of his time telling me that the working classes don't really live they just survive. He was referring to himself and his co-workers, around the table were some nods of agreement – yes that's their 'lot' in life – to survive not really to live.

Every time I come across this type of attitude it shocks me, you'd think I would get used to it wouldn't you, but I don't. I can imagine nothing worse than believing that my life is simply about survival.

I want to take these people to the poorest areas of the third world and compare survival techniques. Would it do any good? I wonder. "Life is either a daring adventure or nothing." We have the power to make it a daring adventure, it doesn't take money, it doesn't take physical muscle power but it does take determination and attitude. These things anyone can have, whether we are tall, short, thin, fat, woman, man, black, white, rich or poor.

Maybe happiness is a lesson that should be taught in schools? How to be happy! How to get excited about things again as we did when we were children!

This same gentleman said that he had to work many hours a week and therefore only had the weekends to get over before it was time to work again. Oh dear, life is ebbing away from that gentleman. When I'm running goal setting sessions with people they often comment "I don't have time to get fit" or "I don't have the money to spend on fancy stuff". Since when did having stuff make us happy? My son gets new stuff every Christmas and the stuff he got last Christmas does not still make him happy next Christmas, I put that down to his age, but it isn't is it? We continue to think that possessions will make us happy.

Our health is one of the most important things, and yet when we collapse in our armchair at the end of the day we pour time into watching programmes on TV. We don't have to go to the gym to get fit; there is enough advice out there on the consumer shelves telling us how to improve our body in just 20 minutes a day.

Why don't we dedicate ourselves to getting fitter and living a little instead of being up to date with the sad lives of people that don't even exist? Be inventive make a 6 inch step and step up and down on it in your own living room. Do one sit up and one press up a day and add on another one every week. Then sit down and work out what else you can do to start living.

Write down here 5 things you used to enjoy doing or that you have fancied having a go at …

1.

2.

3.

4.

5.

Pick the easiest one and write down five ideas for how you can make it happen …

1.

2.

3.

4.

5.

10

Not so bad

✞

"Good Morning – Acme Average Company Limited (obviously all the names have been changed to protect the innocent) How can I help you?" said the monotone voice on the other end of the phone.

"Morning", I said in my usual cheerful way, "How are you?"

There was a pause, I had interrupted her flow – "Not so bad … er … how are you?" she asked more as a knee jerk reaction that an actually enquiry.

"I'm fantastic, thank you"

Breaking the Mirror

"On a Monday!!" she said. "You should work here!!!" The implication being "we'll soon knock that out of you"

It's just a guess but I have a feeling that it wouldn't matter where that lady worked she would say the same thing. Monday morning or no Monday morning; rain or no rain. As soon as we get two consecutive days of sunshine you will hear the complaints of "it's too hot". Unbelievable!

Our behaviour awesome or terrible comes directly from our feelings and emotions, brilliant or otherwise. But we blame the weather, the day of the week, the car breaking down or anything that allows us the luxury of having a moan or just feeling bad. Look out for the grunters, you know the ones, you say "Good Morning" and all they can manage is a grunt. Did you know your feelings and emotions are infectious? Would you want to catch 'Not so bad?'

Imagine for a moment you had a butler (or maid) who came into your room every morning and asked you how you would like to feel that day – would you honestly ask to feel 'not so bad' or 'can't complain', surely not. Maybe we should ask to have a look at the menu "Hmm, let me see now, I'll start with a small glass of 'fantastic', followed by the bowl of 'enthusiastic' and during the day I will raise my game to 'absolutely brilliant', please"

I don't think I ever want to willingly order a not so bad day in my life. But sometimes we end up with it because we haven't considered what we want out of the day first. We have just fallen out of bed into the day and before we know it - it's over.

For the next couple of days listen to the responses you get from asking people how they are. Make a note of some of them below ...

Notice how the different replies made you feel. Obviously it isn't the words that are important but the way in which they are said. But we will cover that kind of thing a bit later. For now just make a note of how others react.

Also, check out how you answer people, find something different to say (preferably something on the positive side) and watch the reactions you get. I love doing that; some people are so used to the standard reply or even a negative one that they don't know how to react.

Quick Recall Session

- When you have even small goals life is very exciting
- Writing down the things you would like to do will increase your chances of getting them done
- Excitement or motivation comes from our hope in the future
- Develop some hope in the future – In other words focus forward not backwards
- Achievement comes from determination
- Desire is essential, if you want to do something enough, you will
- Start with the assumption that it can be done then get to work on the solution
- If they can do it so can you – read stories about people like Helen Keller and don't be amazed be inspired to action
- Decide what you want from the day before you start
- Greet people positively

"People are always blaming their circumstances for what they are. I don't believe in circumstances. The people who get on in this world are the people who get up and look for the circumstances they want, and if they can't find them, make them."

George Bernard Shaw.

11

As Well As They'll Let Me Be

✠

The title of this session comes from a greeting I received from a chap when asking "How are you?" How sad to be so affected by others that it becomes part of our greeting!

Two lawyers were walking down the street on the way to the office. As they approached a newspaper stand one of the lawyers smiled at the vendor. The vendor blanked him. The lawyer then asked to vendor how he was and was once again blanked. The lawyer took a newspaper paid for it and bade the vendor a cheery good day.

The vendor took the money, gave a snort of disgust and muttered something about lawyers that wouldn't bear repeating!!!

The second lawyer turned to the first and said, "Do you always buy from him?" "Oh yes," the first lawyer replied, "and is he always that rude." "Yes, always," he said in a matter of fact kind of way. "Then why," asked the second lawyer, "are you so friendly to him?" The first lawyer turned to his friend and said "Why should I allow his poor behaviour affect mine?"

Sometimes we get caught up in the question of why we should be friendly to others when clearly, the world is becoming a less friendly place, daily.

A better question would be the one that the first lawyer used "why should we let the behaviour of others drag ours down?" Especially when we crave a little bit more happiness and when we know that being cheerful or friendly makes us feel good.

Trying to live to our own standards, without being affected by others can be quite a challenge, but surely it is the proof of great character.

Very much like the statement someone made to me recently: The judge of a person's character is what he would <u>choose</u> to do even if no-one would find out.

Breaking the Mirror

We don't have to lower our standards to the lowest common denominator, even though, it may be an easier route.

One of my friends was walking through a big city and told me that they saw a homeless person selling copies of the magazine 'Big Issue'. It was pouring with rain and everyone was hurrying past. His cry to those who bothered to listen was this, "Big Issue, two free staples with every magazine – transforms into a rain hood."

My friend stopped and bought a copy commenting on his cheerfulness, his reply was, "Why not? I have my problems, so does everyone else, why be miserable too?"

Great advice, being miserable doesn't make our problems go away. So let's focus on what is good around us and maybe, just maybe, things will start to change (but if not at least we won't be miserable too).

On the next page I want you to do an exercise …

Heather Wright

Write down here the names of those closest to you, and next to their names write down the things you like about them. Really focus beyond the irritations and on to the positives …

Breaking the Mirror

When you get good at focussing on what you like about people lets try a more difficult one (or at least for some people it is).

Write down all the good things you can think of about your job, or lack of it …

> Action …
>
> Constantly focus on the good for the next few days. At the end of each day write down the best things that happened to you that day or the thing you liked the best about the day. They don't have to be big things.
>
> Train yourself to notice the good things and then, if you feel you must, we can start to temper it with what some people would call being realistic.

12

Every Day Above Ground is a Good Day

✟

I believe this saying, "every day above ground is a good day," was first coined by a gentleman called W Clement Stone who died in May 2003 having just reached the grand old age of 100. Mr Stone owned and ran a company called Combined Insurance which later became the Aon Corporation.

He started life as a poor kid on the streets of Chicago and become a billionaire and philanthropist. He eventually wrote books and made speeches about being positive; he believed that it was his attitude that made him rich and kept him healthy. I would have to agree with him.

Let's have a look back over the last couple of sections and the things we have covered ...

- ✓ Start with yourself – spend less time blaming others and seek to be alright with yourself first. There will be plenty of time to sort out the rest of the world when you are perfect.

- ✓ Be a yes person – send out yes vibes and you will reap what you sow.

- ✓ Life is about enjoyment, if not what's the point? Start enjoying life (never at the expense of others) and forget about looking stupid.

- ✓ Aim for best behaviour – live excellence and never settle for personal mediocrity.

- ✓ Aim for best behaviour 100% of the time, work excellently, play excellently, rest excellently, give yourself 100% chance to get 100% out.

Breaking the Mirror

Write down three things you are doing differently that are having a positive effect on your life and that of others:

1.

2.

3.

Celebrate over the next couple of days. Celebrate and enjoy being who you are. Aim for excellence and you will achieve more; give more; receive more.

Remember every day above ground is a good day.

13

Be Proactive Instead of Reactive

✢

It is our feelings and emotions which directly affect our behaviour. If we are to change our behaviour we must look to our feelings and emotions. However, we have a tendency to be reactive, when it comes to our feelings.

We get up in the morning and we just happen to feel good or bad. Maybe we blame it on the circumstances such as what the day of the week it is or the weather or the tasks we have to perform that particular day. No wonder we can't expect to feel fantastic all the time if that is the case.

Breaking the Mirror

When we get into our car to go somewhere we rarely get into it and drive aimlessly. We decide where we are going before we even put our coat on. Most of the time we arrive at our destination as planned. If there are road works up ahead we sit and wait until we can get past or we go to enormous lengths to drive round them via all sorts of circuitous routes. We are proactive about where we wish to end up.

Why shouldn't we do the same with our feelings? Before we get up maybe we could spend a moment thinking about what we WANT to do that day and how we WOULD LIKE to feel. Which feelings and emotions will actually assist us in getting the most out of that day?

Ask yourself what behaviour you want from yourself today and then decide how you need to feel in order to achieve that result. When you get up be determined about how you wish to feel. If the fertiliser hits the fan then you may need to take a bit of a detour but feeling lousy about it isn't going to get you to the destination you choose.

Detours can come in all sorts of shapes and sizes; going for a walk in the fresh air can refocus you on your destination, grabbing a quick cup of coffee, reading a section of a positive book or playing some inspiring music. They can all work to get us back on track.

When I was a teenager my friends and I would sit round and play records a lot of the time. The choice of records was determined by how we felt – if we were in a party mood we would play up beat party records, if we were sorrowful because of the demise of a relationship, we would play those sad lost love records.

Let's change it round, I know that when we are down we wish to play down beat music, but it really isn't helpful. Why not do it the other way round? If we need to raise our mood then choose music to give us the mood we need.

Write down some of the negative emotions you suffer from (we all have different habitual emotions) …

In what way do they affect your behaviour?

Have a look back to the behaviours you said were your best and copy them here …

Now, how do you need to feel to produce those behaviours?

Write down some emotions you would like to feel more often …

> Action ...
>
> Over the next day or so pause before you get out of bed, decide how you want to feel before you get up, before you go into the meeting, before you greet the arguing children.

14

Bottling It All Up

✟

Have you ever known someone who appeared to you like a tightly coiled spring and any moment you just know that they will explode?

Maybe it's you and you have exploded at someone at sometime. Some people do this more often and some people do it less often. To some, everything is a crisis but others handle most situations well and then one day for what appears to be no apparent reason, they 'lose it'. There can often be a feeling of relief after letting out all that pent up emotion, but shortly after that, it can be followed by a feeling of remorse or regret.

Because of this, we are told we shouldn't bottle things up, we should let it all out and not allow it to build up. This appears on the surface, like good advice, but not everybody wants to wear their heart on their sleeve.

We must understand that, how we feel about certain situations is not always consistent, nor is it always helpful to share it with others. Most negative emotions are bad for us but yes, I do agree that some can be facilitative and can lead to positive things. However, I have often regretted saying something in the heat of the moment without properly thinking it through and rarely regretted waiting until I was less emotional. In fact often when I wait I find that I don't have the urge to say it anyway.

In a perfect world it would surely be better not to have those negative emotions in the first place. After all positive emotions are great to share (within reason of course) and it's the negative ones that tend to be the most destructive.

In my opinion many of our negative emotions come from dwelling on them rather than from an instant feeling. Something happens and we are convinced that there is a deliberate act of malice or thoughtlessness behind it, we then build on it and justify our negative emotion by having more of them, gathering evidence like an emotional *Miss Marple*. All of this is surely not doing our health, either mentally or physically, any good. In a worse case scenario we start to become neurotic and decide the whole world is conspiring against us.

I was in Australia once running some courses and a young man walked into his university lecture and shot dead several people. He was a foreign student who had trouble standing up to speak in front of people and he was required to present a piece of work to his tutors, he became so obsessed with the idea that they were all against him and would fail him, he shot them. As it turned out he was a straight 'A' student and was to pass the exams with flying colours.

We have all, no doubt, experienced the driver who cuts us up in the traffic. Some days we laugh it off and other days we explode, having irrational thoughts about slashing their tyres or ramming their car up the back, at the time it can seem totally rational, but it isn't.

Over the next couple of days stop yourself dwelling on any negatives.

Start from a point of "What if ..." ie "what if that person has just received some bad news, they are in a hurry and didn't notice me holding the door open?" "What if the other driver is foreign, doesn't know the road system, is in the wrong lane and panicked?" I am sure you can think of a few. Maybe you could make them totally ridiculous so that they make you laugh – laughter is a good emotion when used in the right context.

Think back to a situation in your life when you got angry about something but when you heard the whole story you realised you were wrong. Imagine if you have let out those feelings and then been proved wrong.

15

27,000

✝

We get an average of 27,000 days in our lives. How do you want to remember them?

It's not a massive amount is it?

Whose permission are we waiting for to enjoy ourselves or to start feeling good about ourselves? I have heard people saying … "just wait until the kids grow up" … "until they leave college" … "until I have paid off my mortgage" … "until I have retired" … until, until, until.

What a waste.

We strive to earn enough money to go on holiday or pay off the mortgage. We forget to live today because we are focussed so much on the future.

Have you noticed that when there is a death in the family, none of these things matter as much anymore? Obviously we need to temper our living for today, selling the house today and blowing the lot on the next horse race is ultimate short-termism, but then waiting all your life for retirement is the opposite.

The goals we have need to be long, medium and short term. Each day needs to have goals. They may be as simple as aiming for great feelings, greeting everyone we meet in a shockingly positive manner or ending the day with as much energy as we started it.

My favourite is to make a positive difference to as many people as I can that day, doing things for people that will make their life a little better or easier, even if they never find out I did it.

What would you like people to say about you when you aren't around? Imagine that you are standing reading a notice board and round the corner from you are a group of people who know you and they don't know you are there. What would you like them to say about you?

Breaking the Mirror

Write it down below ...

How much difference is there between the reality and the desire?

Heather Wright

What can you practically do differently, over the next couple of days that, will affect the way people think about you? (Bringing it more in line with what you would like them to say about you). Write down below something you intend to do differently ...

Breaking the Mirror

Imagine for the next couple of days that you are in the middle of a test. You are being tested on your unswerving ability to keep your feelings and emotions positive. Everything that is thrown at you over the next couple of days will be deliberately designed to catch you out. Don't let it. Stick to it and stick to your plan for doing something different.

Write down how you get on below ...

Quick Recall Session

- Don't let other people's attitude drag yours down
- It's bad enough that things go wrong without feeling bad about it too
- Every day above ground is indeed a good day
- Learn to celebrate – even small things
- Decide how you want to feel each day and aim for it no matter what
- Forgive yourself when you don't achieve it and start again – it's no big deal
- Don't bottle it up – work on feeling better instead
- Find something good to think about
- We get an average of 27,000 days and only one chance to make the most of it
- Today is tomorrow's yesterday - how do you want to remember it?
- Be aware of how your feelings affect your behaviour – aim for great feelings and the behaviour will follow
- Consciously be proactive, not reactive, about what you expect from each day

Breaking the Mirror

"The world is a looking-glass, and gives back to every man the reflection of his own face. Frown at it, and it will in turn look sourly upon you; laugh at it and with it and it is a jolly kind companion ..."

William Makepeace Thackeray, Vanity Fair.

16

It's a Choice

✝

Everyone talks about attitudes nowadays. We even throw it at our children when their tone displeases us, "Watch that attitude!" Or we hear people say, "You've got to have a positive attitude." People say it often, without really thinking or knowing, what a truly positive attitude is. Most people mean that you've always got to look on the bright side of life. Ignore the bad and glibly pretend everything is great. Is that what a positive attitude really is?

Two men looked out of prison bars,
One saw mud, the other saw stars.

There are two types of attitude, a negative one and a positive one. A negative one sees all the problems, especially the insurmountable ones, it lacks trust, it is a puppet to circumstance, and it thinks life is mostly about what happens to us. The positive one is not glib blind positivity. The positive attitude sees the problems but views them as learning experiences. It does not trust blindly but it is aware that, although some things cannot be taken at face value, why assume the worst before it has actually happened.

A positive attitude is about planning and goal setting, it is about persistence and commitment, it is about the way we treat others and the way we treat ourselves on the inside.

Most people do not fail; most people give up or do not attempt things in the first place. Our attitude is a choice every day. We make that choice unconsciously and when circumstances hit us we choose our attitude towards that circumstance. It is very often a knee jerk reaction. When the fertiliser hits the fan what sort of behaviour do you need? Best or worst?

Therefore what sort of feelings do you need? Great or terrible? So what sort of attitude generates the feelings you need and therefore the behaviour you must have.

Which attitude leads to creativity and dogged determination?

What current negative facts/circumstances do you have in your life?

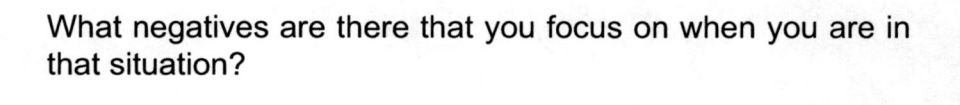

What negatives are there that you focus on when you are in that situation?

What positives can you find in that situation? (This can be a tough one but give it a go).

Life is all about attitudes towards the facts. Think about times in the past when you have overcome something by determination. What can you learn from it?

Breaking the Mirror

> Action ...
>
> Watch the people around you over the next few days. Spot the ones who choose a negative attitude versus those who choose a positive one.

17

Blame Cultures

✠

Blame is a tough one to deal with; from very early in our lives we learn to point the finger. Often, we don't really care in which direction we are pointing it, as long as it isn't at ME!!

The motivational negatives of blame hit home to me about six months ago. One of the chaps from work asked to borrow my relatively new car to go to a sales meeting. Of course I obliged and when he returned I was interested in how his sales meeting had gone. He was pretty sheepish as he crept into the office and instead of telling me about the meeting he informed me that he had 'bumped' my car. I could tell by his face that he was feeling pretty awful about this, there was no need for me to get angry, so in order to make him feel better about it I hardly paid it any attention and continued to ask about the meeting. Eventually I turned back to my computer to continue the work I was doing but he insisted that I go outside to assess the damage. He had reversed into a post of some sort and the damage eventually cost quite a considerable sum. However apart from allowing me to vent my anger, blaming him would have been pointless, so I didn't bother. I just patted him on the shoulder and told him not to worry.

At this point he praised my attitude and said he was impressed with the way I had lived my espoused values. During the next few days I deliberately didn't mention the damage to anyone; I didn't even tease or joke about it. A couple of weeks later my car was being repaired for a few days and a courtesy car was not available (I was in too much of a hurry to wait).

During the time I was car-less I got lifts from anyone available and borrowed cars when I could from whoever was around. Thankfully I eventually received that wonderful telephone call that said my car would be ready the next day. After replacing the handset I announced to whoever was listening, "I get my car back tomorrow, I will be so glad when I get it back," at which one of my colleagues retorted "We'll all be glad when you get your car back!" My next comment was a knee jerk reaction, no thought behind it, just purely defensive emotional response. "Well, It wasn't my fault."

Half way through the sentence my brain kicked in and I realised what I was saying. A quick look at the guy who had bumped my car confirmed that, in a split second, I had just undone all the carefully considered work I had done for the previous weeks. His shoulders had slumped and the back of his neck had gone bright red.

The blame effect is like a set of dominoes that knock down a long line or like the black spot in Treasure Island that everyone wants to get rid of as quickly as possible and pass on to someone/anyone else. Just so long as they are not left with it.

Those who have a negative attitude look for someone or something to blame, "It's not my fault," "It's too complicated," "I never had the right background/education/parents." etc.

All this does is make us feel better about being negative, it doesn't take us forward to a better place or to better behaviour, in fact it can then lead to a downward spiral and take us backwards.

Listen to the people around you for obvious blame phrases, but then listen out for the more subtle implied blame, "what did you do that for?" and other such phrases. Then ask yourself why they said it – it may be a genuine question or a need to know, in order to move forward or is it the one used more often to find someone to blame, maybe to take the heat off ourselves.

Find a better way of asking questions like these ...

"Who took the pen from my desk?"

"Which stupid idiot left the back door unlocked last night? We could have been murdered in our beds!!"

"What did you do that for?"

Become aware of how often those around you blame someone else or a fact for a negative outcome.

18

It's Not the Facts

✞

Life can be tough sometimes can't it? There are things that happen to us that seem totally out of our control. When that happens there are usually a series of things that happen one after the other and it feels like we are on the roller coaster from hell and there is no stopping to get off.

I remember the time when I was first introduced to this type of thinking or philosophy, it was summer and shortly after I learnt about it we went on holiday to Cornwall. Cornwall is a beautiful place; I certainly find it peaceful visiting the little towns hidden in the nooks and crannies of the British coastline. However, you can never forget that this is Britain and glorious sunshine is not guaranteed.

One day during our holiday, the weather was less than wonderful; in fact it was raining and cold. After sitting inside looking out at the rain for sometime, one of my friends piped up, "Heather, you're into positive thinking … make the sun shine!" Now, I know it was a flippant throw away comment but that isn't what it is about at all.

Stuff happens, some of it is good, some of it is neutral and some of it is bad, occasionally some of it is disastrous. I wonder how many events or facts have been absolutely disastrous for you in the end.

Arthur Ashe was interviewed many times in his career but I have heard of one interview he gave after contracting AIDS. He was asked "Do you ever ask "why ME?" His reply was astonishing, he said, "No, because if I ask why me for all the bad things that happen in my life, I will have to ask why me for all the great things too and I don't want to do that."

Bad stuff happens; it happens to all of us. I agree that some people seem to have more than their fair share, but sitting around feeling sorry for ourselves just lengthens it, adds to it and certainly doesn't change it. Our primary reaction is often negative, understandably so, but we can relearn that and teach ourselves a different reaction just as we can relearn something physically.

Ask yourself this question –

When the fertiliser hits the fan what sort of behaviour do you need, best or worst? (Remember our descriptions of what we are like at our best)

I must assume, you have answered 'best', in which case we must have feelings and emotions that will lead to it. In order to have those great feelings, that will lead to best behaviour, what sort of attitude to we need to choose in order to give us great feelings and thus lead to fantastic behaviours?

So, what is a positive attitude?

Does it mean we skip about and ignore the negatives?

Absolutely not, we must be aware of them, but we need to view them in the perspective of the outcome we desire. A negative attitude looks at the situation and says "Oh no, look where I am, how depressing, isn't life hard?" A positive attitude says "how can I achieve my goal even though this thing has happened?"

This is not as some may think, blind positivity, instead, it is thinking of solutions rather than the problem, it is looking forward instead of looking back. We do not wish to walk into the future facing backwards.

Positive people have reasons why they must get to where they want to be. Negative people have excuses for why they haven't and why they can't. They are often so caught up in the facts that they can't see where they could be going.

The weird thing is that the excuses and the reasons can often be identical.

Right now I would bet that there is someone living in the roughest neighbourhood you can imagine; drugs, violence, alcohol abuse and illness may infest their lives on a daily basis and they will stay there believing that they have no choice.

Equally there will be someone else in that same environment, who will believe that they must get out and they couldn't possibly stay there, maybe they have a dream or a goal; perhaps they have met someone who has given them the spark of self belief or an idea which is growing inside them. One day they will look back and say to themselves "look what I did, look where I came from."

Same circumstances – different attitude.

Heather Wright

What excuses do you hear people use?

Do you have any that you use?

How could you turn these around?

19

Being Impressive

✜

There is nothing impressive about having a positive attitude when everything is going right. The impressive thing is being positive when things aren't going so well or even when things are terrible.

Maybe now would be a good time to decide just what we mean by a positive attitude. Let's start with the definition of what it isn't.

It isn't - plastering a smile on your face when your partner has just left you, your son is in jail, and your teenage daughter just came home and told you she is pregnant, your house is being repossessed and you haven't a penny in your pocket to buy food for your next meal.

It isn't - being an irritation to everyone else by spouting inane platitudes at every opportunity.

It isn't - ignoring other people's pain and sorrow, when they need sympathy, by making them feel guilty about their emotions.

However ...

It is - a sense of determination that when everything uncontrollable goes negative we can still deal with the controllables and focus on our destination.

It is - where we want to be and how we are going to get there; rather than falling back into a sense of being a victim and having no control over anything.

It is - leading by example and choosing appropriate and meaningful illustrations to share with those who may require a boost.

It is – knowing that everyone does not feel the same at the same time and that timing is essential. By using this knowledge, we can maintain others' trust in our opinions, knowing when they need that shoulder to cry on and when they are ready for a gentle push in a positive direction.

It is – learning to balance, forgiving yourself for occasional lapses and striving for constant improvement.

It is – an easy to explain philosophy and a tough mental discipline.

It is – a logical way to overcome emotional challenges.

It is – accepting responsibility for the things that happen and therefore for the journey to where you wish to be.

Over the next couple of pages make a list of the things that prevent you from being at your best and getting to where you want to be.

Now consider them carefully, which of these things are definitely uncontrollable. E.g. bad weather, traffic jams etc. Place a cross beside them.

What about the controllables? Place a tick beside those and write down some ideas about how you can overcome them (any ideas will do – just brain storm it).

Think of these things over the next few days and come up with some more ideas. Once you get good at sorting out the uncontrollables from the controllables you will be able to look at the uncontrollables and decide how you may be able to get round those too.

For example ...

People who suffer from S.A.D. (seasonal affective disorder) because of bad weather – plan for some time in the sun (or, carefully, on a sun bed) every six months.

Traffic jams – listen to positive attitude tapes when stuck, take detours or the more expensive option, purchase a Satellite Navigation system.

There is always a way.

20

24/7

✞

I bumped into an old acquaintance the other week. I was not sure whether I felt better or worse after I spoke to her. By rights she should be a huge success in life (and by success I mean it in every sense of the word), she studied and received all the correct qualifications, she started a splendid career, she has determination and is a strong character.

But (you knew there was going to be a BUT didn't you) she can't hold down a job, her relationships are a mess and her life is going nowhere. What is wrong? I have thought about it long and hard and I have a pretty good idea what it is: Values and attitude.

This person has always lived with an attitude of "what can I get away with?" In other words, how many sick days can I pull off before they get suspicious? How much can I claim for on the insurance? If I travel second class can I claim expenses for first class? It's an attitude; some would say it is a set of values, whichever it is; it seriously limits our ability to be of value to others.

I can't find any irrefutable scientific proof, but there is a universal or maybe moral law that says everything we do that is negative – whether to a person or a nameless entity - detracts from our self concept. The reverse is also true, it is impossible to raise someone else's self esteem, without raising your own.

My children have many board games and often they are games that try to emulate real life. One may pick a card which says "You give some money to charity move on three paces" or "You win a Nobel Peace Prize take 10 happiness points." In real life, we don't always get our rewards immediately; sometimes the rewards we get don't show in obvious ways.

I can't help thinking that the Ten Commandments weren't given to us as a set of rules to beat us with but instead as a set of guidelines for living in harmony, more like a parent acting in despair of squabbling children, sick of them constantly making each other unhappy.

In an interview Paul McCartney was once asked about his charitable works; I think the interviewer was trying to imply that because we never hear much about it that he doesn't do much. His answer was superb "If you heard about them they wouldn't be charity, they would be marketing". I think he picked up the card which said "You give to charity move on three paces, if you do it secretly move on six paces."

My husband and I have been through some rough times (business-wise/financially) and during one such time a friend must have heard about how bad things were. So one night, there was a ring at our front door and when I answered, three or four bags of shopping had been left on the door step. Every now and again we contemplate about who it was and we have narrowed it down, but to be really honest I hope we never find out, because our debt is currently to anyone who needs our help.

When you live with a great attitude others have a great attitude back. Negative attitudes also return to haunt us. A fantastic attitude does not necessarily mean outstanding wealth, total happiness and a life spanning four generations, but you definitely stand more of a chance.

Heather Wright

What things have you done that are self-less? (It's OK this book is for your eyes only)

What things could you do?

> **Action ...**
>
> Look round for opportunities to act selflessly and help someone else over the next couple of days and enjoy the buzz purely for the sake of enjoying the buzz.

Quick Recall Session

- Attitude is a choice 100% of the time
- It's not the facts themselves that make us feel bad but our attitudes towards them
- Blame is a subtle knife cutting away at people's self esteem and trust
- Pause before you point the finger
- Stuff happens – get over it
- Don't waste time finding excuses; look for reasons why you must
- Be impressive – stand out from the crowd – look for solutions when everyone else is staring at the problem
- Things are either controllable or uncontrollable, let's not waste time moaning about the uncontrollable, be busy sorting out the controllables
- Sort out what values you want to live by and stick to them
- Great attitudes and fantastic values shine out of every pore and affect the outcome of things even when you're not trying

"Strange as it may seem, life becomes serene and enjoyable precisely when selfish pleasures and personal success are no longer the guiding goals."

Mihaly Csikszentmihalyi, Psychologist and Educator.

21

It's a Way of Life

✞

Let's take it one step further. Recently, at a session for CEO's (Chief Executive Officers) a gentleman confessed to me and all the others present, that he had always made a note of everyone who had wronged him in some way. He then waited for an opportunity to find a way to return their perceived evil deed, even letting them know, that it was his deliberate act that had made them suffer.

After we had all spoken about attitudes, he decided that he was not going to do this anymore, which is quite a turn around. Even better than this, he said that he was going to get out his 'little black book', take everyone in it out to lunch or dinner and let them know that they were

Breaking the Mirror

henceforth not on the list. I couldn't believe it, what a change of heart, and he was totally sincere.

That is definitely a case of going the extra mile. Sometimes it takes something extra to get it out of our system. Going the extra mile can become a habit, a positive habit, to get into.

Why should I? Before I give you my reasons – why don't you write below, in what way you think going the extra mike, would benefit you. And if your answer is "it wouldn't!" then try to imagine what someone else might say if they were to recommend it to you.

Well, my first answer is to refer back to that last couple of sessions about life philosophy and getting exactly what you give in life.

My second answer is about adding value. If we get into the habit of going the extra mile for people in general our brains become more creative about how to add value all the time. This in turn adds to our general worth as an employee primarily but also as a partner, friend and or colleague.

We need to give people a reason to employ us, promote us or give us a pay rise and if this philosophy is not appreciated where we are, then there are plenty of jobs for those who add value to a company.

Adding value is about doing that bit extra above and beyond what we are expected to do. It is only possible to do this if we are achieving our current targets, there is no value in someone who doesn't do what they are paid to do, but can list the many triumphs of tasks they have completed that they have not been asked to do!!!!

Imagine for a moment what a difference it would make to you, if those who have most impact on your life also took up this challenge, what would added value mean to you? It doesn't take a lot does it? I doubt very much if you have just had your head flooded with impossible unachievable ideas. I certainly know that if my children

Breaking the Mirror

not only did their homework promptly when they arrived through the door, but then also cleared and laid the table for dinner without being asked, it would make life that little bit more comfortable. Obviously at their young ages I don't expect that to happen straight away but it is something for them to aim for.

List below the people you have most contact with and write beside their names a couple of things you could do to go that extra distance. Remembering that I am not encouraging you to be a 'push over' – it is still OK to say no, in fact you will feel alright about saying no when you need to, when you feel you are doing something elsewhere.

Heather Wright

Appreciation of others when they do this is also important.

List below things you have noticed others doing either for you or for someone else (some of these maybe very small but are none the less important) …

22

Beliefs

✝

So, we are often told to have a positive attitude, but very few people tell us how. Besides, attitude is a symptom of something else, an attitude positive or otherwise is the product of our beliefs; our beliefs about ourselves, our beliefs about others, our beliefs about our culture or even our beliefs about the world in general.

The strange thing is that we are not born with any beliefs. I feel disinclined to argue nature versus nurture as no-one will ever win that argument. No-one will ever prove that you have a temper like your father because you were born with your father's temper genes or because you have been told all of your life that "you have a temper like your father's!!" I have seen copious amounts of studies done on twins separated at birth and twins not separated at birth, identical twins and non identical twins and some prove one thing and some prove the other.

The most important point is surely, if you have a temper like your father's – can you change it should you so desire? I hope to shed more light on that question as we move through this book together.

For now, let's just deal with the beliefs we have, genetic or not. Largely we can put our beliefs into two separate categories - **'limiting beliefs'** and **'inspiring beliefs'**.

Limiting beliefs are the ones which drive the negative attitude and therefore all the excuses. "I believe I can't do anything about this situation, therefore I will have a negative attitude towards it, with the excuse that it's not my fault – this will lead to terrible feelings and emotions and thus poor behaviour." All this can be summed up in two very simple words "I can't."

On the other hand we have **inspiring beliefs** that tell us that there is always a way to do anything, all we have to do is find that way. The belief that we can do something, even if it may take us a long time or include a large amount of effort, leads to a brilliant attitude towards whatever 'fact' (remember section 18 – It's not the facts it's how you react) it is that we are contemplating, followed by great feelings and emotions and thus the potential of our best behaviour – I like to sum this up with the words "How can I?"

This simple question opens up the brain or mind to its more creative side and doesn't leave room for that inner voice to contradict a glib statement like "I can" with "liar, liar, pants on fire" which I tend to find my inner voice quietly singing away to me deep down.

Spend some time now listing some of your limiting beliefs down one side of next page and down the other side list some of your inspiring beliefs. They don't have to be all about you but they do have to be beliefs that affect you in some way.

For example, the belief that the government will never change their policy on people who work in glass blowing factories not being allowed to blow more than three dozen glasses a day (in case you haven't guessed it, I made this one up!!), will only affect you if you work in that area and is therefore only limiting to those people.

Got it? I'm sure you have.

Limiting	Inspiring

Breaking the Mirror

Keep noticing beliefs over the next few days – you will hear people often give themselves away with little throw away comments.

Jot a few down that you hear ...

23

More on Beliefs

✣

Where do our beliefs come from? If we aren't born with any beliefs, from where did that one about, "I'm no good at foreign languages" come? After all, when you were a baby you weren't born English speaking, French speaking or Chinese speaking. As a matter of fact I have a friend who has adopted a beautiful little girl from China, she came over here as a baby, she is now four or five and she doesn't speak Chinese!!

The skill of speaking was taught to you as you grew and if you had, as have many people before, moved from one country to another and thus been surrounded by a different language you may now speak more than one. A gentleman I was speaking to the other day, has a daughter of aged 11, who currently speaks somewhere in the region of 4 languages fluently and three more partially (and I suspect that when he says 'partially' he is being modest on her behalf).

Is it the same for all of our beliefs? Who can say? One thing we can be pretty sure of is that some things come easier than others, but if we work at the others and find a way to learn that suits us, we can pick up just about most things. One of the biggest factors must be our desire to do so.

When we are still young, while our brains are at their most malleable, the adults around us, whom we trust to be experts, tell us what we are like. They say "you're clumsy," "he's not a morning person" or "what a determined child you are." Sometimes we even implant these ideas for the sake of humour, for example, "here comes trouble," "we call him the terminator" or "she's going to be the boss when she grows up." At this age, when the child is looking for an identity, perhaps we need to be more careful about how we chose to project our opinions onto them.

What I am trying to say is that all children spill drinks but constant reinforcing of the fact will only make matters worse. My brother was so clumsy my mother said he could walk into an empty room and fall over. Her answer was to send him (and me) to ballet lessons (I hated them), he loved them and ended up at the Royal Ballet School, which was the top ballet school in the world at that time.

Listen to conversations around you for the next couple of days, watch out for statements about behaviour which label people rather than talk about their behaviour, for example "he's clumsy" rather than "that was a careless thing to do."

Describe yourself …

Which of these words you have used are factual and which are beliefs that you have developed over time.

Which beliefs would you like to change?

> Action ...
>
> Concentrate on your inspiring beliefs, focus on them, write them on small cards and place them where you will see them – e.g. on the inside of your car visor, as a screen saver on your computer, stuck to your bathroom mirror or on the fridge door.

24

Even More on Beliefs

☦

Beliefs can limit or inspire us whether they are based on fact or fiction. The only difference is that, because they are our beliefs, we would always argue that our belief is fact. I am constantly surprised by how many times we make assumptions that, because it is so for us, it must be the same for others. I heard someone talking the other day about something they had done and when someone asked why they had done it the response was "well, you do, don't you?" Maybe it makes us feel better if we believe we are not alone in our beliefs. Maybe we think that, the more people who believe the same, the more it becomes a concrete fact.

On the 6th of May 1954 Roger Bannister ran a mile in less than 4 minutes.

It was an amazing achievement, even more so when one considers that before he did it, the belief of the doctors of that day, was that if anyone achieved this particular feat, they would actually die. If their lungs didn't collapse and they didn't have a heart attack then their brain would die of oxygen starvation and that would definitely kill them.

I don't know about you, but I think those are three pretty good reasons to simply be one of the officials on the sidelines cheering Roger on! However, the doctors were wrong and Roger, (who was also a doctor) was thankfully still alive when he finished the race. There were hundreds of people who had the skill level to achieve this feat at the time of Mr Bannister, one of whom was John Landis, who achieved it less than a month after Roger – less than a month too late.

I often wonder if John Landis would have achieved it, if the belief that it was possible hadn't already been changed or if the 200 people who achieved it in the next two years would have succeeded, if Roger Bannister hadn't changed their beliefs.

Then there is Vasiliy Alekseyev the Russian Super Heavy Weight Lifting Champion who in the 1970's Alekseyev was unchallenged and set 80 world records. However there comes a time, even in a champion's life, when a coach has to push an athlete even higher than he or she believes they can go. As he approached the Olympics, his coaches felt he needed to go one step further than before to ensure his continued success, so they tried to persuade him to try for 600kg (a cumulative total of three lifts).

Every training session they would ask him to try. He would try and he would fail stating that 600 kilos was impossible and would never be achieved by anyone. His coaches would never finish on a negative note they would make him lift his current record lift, before finishing his training session, so that he was in a positive frame of mind to try again next session.

Two weeks before the Olympics, his coaches had to confess to him that all along both sets of weights were identical and he had therefore been successfully lifting an "impossible" weight for weeks, in the belief that it was only his current achievable weight.

In the 1972 and 1976 Olympics, Alekseyev's combined lifts, earned him the gold medal and further records.

Although these two examples are physical ones, how much more can we break the chains of our mental limitations, by changing our beliefs about ourselves?

Have a look through the newspapers over the next few days – spot some stories that show someone's beliefs limiting them or inspiring them, or maybe about them changing their beliefs in order to achieve something they wanted. Make a note of the stories you have seen below, cut them out and stick them somewhere prominent.

25

Conditioning or "if you do what you've always done, you'll get what you always got"

☦

Psychologists tell us that our beliefs come from our conditioning. That is, everything that has happened to us, from the moment we were born (and maybe even the nine months before that). Many argue over how much of our character, personality and therefore conditioning we are already born with. I find it difficult to imagine anyone ever winning the nature versus nurture argument.

I also believe that our self concept and our personality are different but I find it very hard to believe that God would give us a personality that is harmful to ourselves or others. However if a child is predisposed to be single minded, then because of the conditioning it is exposed to, it may become an adult who is focussed on success in business, determined to change the world for the good of others or even become a dictator, willing to commit genocide to achieve their own ambitions.

It has often been said that the line between genius and psychopathic behaviour is a fine one, like the drive to do good turns into an obsession and is used for evil.

I have been told in the past that we are born with two fears – the fear of falling and the fear of loud noises, the first supposedly generated by the birth experience and the latter by the fact that we have spend 9 months in a quiet environment and we suddenly arrive in this noisy world.

Who are we to argue, I have never successfully interviewed a baby in my life, even having had two of my own I was never sure whether the cry they were emitting was a hungry cry, a bored cry or a "get this nappy pin out of my butt" cry.

Our conditioning is the result of experience, culture, gender, parents, siblings, peers, teachers, the media and much, much more. The media influence is one that always fascinates me. It is very difficult to untangle the beliefs we have developed by ourselves versus those into which the media have had some input. In today's society it must surely be one of the biggest influences. My children have nightmares influenced by television programmes; they have knowledge of how to deal with vampires and zombies (probably better than they know how to cross the road safely). It is certainly difficult to imagine a world in which there is no media influence.

Even if a family chooses not to possess a television or to read the newspapers, one would have to cut oneself off from everyone else, in order not to be affected. We look at news items about Third World Countries where citizens are fed only the propaganda of their present government and wonder how they can believe such 'lies', but I often wonder how much of the media coverage from which we develop our opinions, are totally factual?

This is not a speech against the media it's just curiosity on my part, after all the only reason newspapers are full of negative press is because that's what sells.

Enough of this; we must also acknowledge the effect that genetics has on our conditioning as well as on our health. However I believe that, the biggest influence on our own conditioning and therefore on us, is ourselves.

Our conditioning may have started the process off, but we exacerbate it by repeating it to ourselves, albeit internally.

It isn't the experience, its <u>how</u> we choose to think about it that matters. I agree that the way we think about it may be the product of previous conditioning, but once we get to the age of reasoning (whatever age that may be) we have a choice regarding the way we think. Do we want to continuously follow the path we have been travelling down with which we are not totally happy? or do we wish to try something different.

Remember: if we keep doing the same things we have always done we will get what we have always got. In order to <u>get</u> something different we must <u>do</u> something different.

It astounds me how many people moan daily about their lot in life, but if you try to persuade them to do something different, they will argue against it as though their life depends upon it.

How many times do you find yourself arguing against something just because it makes you uncomfortable or maybe even a bit scared?

Listen to your conversations and those of others and note down how many discussions are actually based on emotions rather than logic.

Try to look beyond what the people are saying and notice why they are actually saying it.

Make notes below …

Quick Recall Session

- This is a life philosophy – 24 hours a day, 7 days a week, not a jacket to put on when necessary
- Aim to go the extra mile just for the sake of it
- Our beliefs drive our attitude good or otherwise
- In order to achieve our best we must have inspiring beliefs
- We weren't born with any beliefs, they were developed and can therefore be re-developed, in favour of where and who we want to be
- Focus on your inspiring beliefs and those of others
- Our beliefs don't have to be based on fact to affect us, we just think they are
- Our beliefs are built by our conditioning
- Above all else our conditioning = our thoughts
- We can choose what to think in order to achieve the beliefs and thus the attitude that dictates our feelings, which manifests in our behaviour.

Breaking the Mirror

"I think the thing I keep saying to myself every year ... is that I want to become a better player at the end of the year than I was at the beginning ... If I can keep doing that year after year for the rest of my career, I'll have a pretty good career."

Tiger Woods, Professional Golfer.

26

It's the Thought That Counts

✢

After we have got over the shock of realising that it is our thoughts that are affecting the way we behave and there is no-one else to blame really, there is also a sense of excitement of how much we can achieve, knowing that we have only to change the way we think in order to 'go for it', so to speak.

Our biggest challenge is that we learn more from our negative conditioning than from our positive conditioning. This is because of our 'fight or flight' mechanism and is there to keep us alive. Obviously if we learn from our negatives and because of this, our adverse reactions become faster then we have more of a chance to keep ourselves alive in the dangerous world we evolved in; but because of this it takes more positives to overcome a negative. If we add this to the fact that, during our lifetime we often receive more negatives than we do positives and on top of that we perceive that we receive more negatives and less positives than we probably actually do, it is no small wonder that we are more likely to develop a negative habit of thinking than a positive one.

It is very tempting to spend a great deal of time on why we became the person we are now. To be really honest I am more interested in where we are going than where we have come from. If we walk backwards into the future (ie if we spend all our lives looking back) we will not achieve what we would wish to achieve and are actually more likely to paralyse ourselves with fear than facilitate any sort of progress.

No-one else can control the way we think.

How fantastic is that!!

It is possible to be manipulated so we must learn to overcome the negative conditioning around us and choose to think in a way that moves us towards the behaviours we want to see more of and away from those behaviours that we would prefer to get rid of.

We are often told that those who achieve more in life are the ones who have goals and this is no doubt true. It amazes me how few people set themselves goals on a regular basis. Within the sphere of the people who set goals, the most successful ones are those who concentrate on the behaviours they need in order to become the person they need to become and thus to achieve their goals.

What goals do you have right now?

Over the next few pages I want you to write them down – some of them may be large goals, some may be small daily or medium monthly goals.

Just write them all down and then you can put them into an order that makes sense to you. If you can't think far ahead, write down a couple of short term ones.

Short Term (During the next few months) …

Heather Wright

Medium Term (Within the next year or two) ...

Long Term (5-10 years) ...

Heather Wright

Absolutely Massive Ones (Things you dream about that you would secretly love to be a reality) ...

27

Tough Lessons

✝

These can be hard lessons to learn. So let's go back over it again. Our behaviour is driven by our feelings and emotions. Great feelings and emotions driving the behaviour we like and want more of, terrible feelings driving the behaviour we would rather forget about but unfortunately creeps up on us, when we would rather it went away.

Our feelings and emotions come from our attitude towards the facts around us and not, as we like to think, from the facts themselves. Our attitude is determined by our beliefs whether they be limiting or inspiring.

Inspiring beliefs lead to determination and a persistence that will overcome as many obstacles as we need to reach our end goal.

Strong self belief gives us the ability to spot opportunities and turn them to our advantage and allows us to learn from our mistakes instead of berating ourselves. It enables us to forgive others instead of blaming them.

Finally, it is our conditioning that builds our beliefs and above everything else that conditions us, it is our thoughts that condition us the most. An event may only happen once but we can think about that event time and again; it is our choice which things we spend time with in our heads; it is our choice how we decide to think about things.

Instead of being reactive to the events around us, it is more productive to ask ourselves "Is this train of thought helpful?" "Do these thoughts lead to the sort of behaviour I want to have?"

The one thing we have total control over is our mind. It is possible to learn how to think. It is possible to choose how to think in a more productive manner instead of just allowing our thoughts to build negative beliefs about us.

I would like you to consider the following question:

"What would you dare to attempt if you knew you couldn't fail?"

Write it down. Try to be specific ...

Now write down the type of people, you think, could achieve it? (Whatever it is)

What sort of behaviours do those type of people display?

Which of these behaviours do you think that, with a bit of work, you could develop? Write it all down. Just dump it down on the paper. Don't try to second guess yourself.

28

Daazen Matta Eets Een De Past

☦

I sometimes find it difficult to understand why we feel the need to dwell on the negatives in our past. A need to find an excuse for our failing's maybe? Or a reason not to have to try when our belief is that we are going to fail?

We have so much ahead of us if we would only look to our future. Maybe just spending time with the present would be a good start for many!!

I love to use the example used in "The Lion King", there is a moment in the film when the wise old baboon hits the young Lion over the head with a stick. After rubbing his head the lion asks "What did you do that for?" and the answer is given, "Daazen matta eets een de past" roughly translated as, it doesn't matter it's in the past.

What a simple but well illustrated way of moving on. I know that some events in our lives need to be looked at but only for the purpose of being able to learn from them.

To prevent ourselves falling into the same traps again, or to unlock some secret meaning that may help give us the push we need to stride with confidence into a better future.

My husband has been accused of hiding his problems from people who supposedly want to help him. He, however, is an extremely together kind of guy and deals with his problems as and when they occur and then moves on. In this way he carries a minimal amount of baggage around with him.

Let's not assume that there always has to be something wrong. Keep your eyes on what you want in life instead of constantly looking back and saying "ooooo that was painful." Learn from it and move on. The process of learning from something does not have to be long and drawn out although sometimes the lesson may hit you at a later date. Let it go. You do not have to be driven by the negatives, constantly reminded of your failings and bad experiences, you can be anything you want to be.

Heather Wright

In the days of high internet use I get many meaningful saying and stories sent to me. Here's one I liked and made a note of, see what you think …

As we travel down life's highways
Keep your eyes upon the goal
Focus on the doughnut
And not upon the hole

… it may not be profound, but it works.

What things have you been sitting on from your past that you return to every now and again to relive and dwell upon? Maybe they are only triggered by the presence of a particular individual.

Write down your thoughts on it below …

Now decide to let it go, get rid of it and write down the benefits of letting go of it …

Practise letting go for the next few days; keep saying it to yourself – it's in the past, forget it.

29

Forgiveness

✟

National Forgiveness Day – have you ever heard of anything so stupid? A day of people forgiving each other on a national scale? Actually, come to think of it, it's a great idea. Bitterness and jealousy are debilitating emotions.

However, there are some emotions that can, under the right circumstances facilitate positive action.

Anger is one of these emotions. To get angry about the injustice of a situation can inspire us to do something that will move us on. In fact many changes in law and policies, such as Women's Rights, Anti-apartheid and many more have obviously been driven by people who at some time have got so angry about the status quo that they have become passionate enough to take action.

Fear is another emotion that I would not recommend as a long term part of our lives, because to live in fear can only be destructive and can sap our resolve the majority of the time. However fear of fire has driven individuals from burning buildings and fear of failure has driven many an entrepreneur to creative action.

But, I have rarely seen jealousy and bitterness as facilitating emotions. In today's society where the divorce rate is high there are many bitter ex-partners. They walk around hating, harbouring thoughts of revenge, nurturing their mental wounds; some are even on a constant search for a friendly ear in which to pour out their sceptic words.

Many a child has suffered at the hands of two people who are so busy fighting each other that they cannot see the damage they are doing to those caught in the fall out.

Maybe its time for you to forgive someone today! "Why should I?" "They don't deserve it!" "Look at what they did" or "You couldn't possibly understand" are some of the words that come out when forgiveness is mentioned.

You may be absolutely right but I can't find anything positive that comes from not forgiving them. Forgiveness doesn't mean giving in to every demand and making ourselves a doormat. It doesn't mean that there aren't any consequences of the negative actions. For example, if a child does something they have been told not to do and they say sorry, then forgiveness does not mean that they don't get grounded or have to pay for the thing they broke. Forgiveness is about putting the emotion aside.

It is OK to say "I forgive you, I am no longer angry, you are still going to have to pay for the vase you broke but you are forgiven," or "I forgive you for lying to me, its in the past now, it will take some time to build up my trust again."

For me forgiveness is about stopping the negative emotion from eating away at us. In many cases the bitterness causes us more harm than the person it is aimed at. It causes us to make decisions that may not be the best ones and can turn a grown adult back into a playground child. For our own sake it is time to get over it, to move on, to allow our wounds to heal.

For some of us the forgiveness may need to be turned inward, maybe it is time to forgive yourself, none of us is perfect. We all make mistakes; give yourself a break.

A large number of people recite The Lord's Prayer, whether they are a devout Christian or not. For those of you who can be even occasionally caught doing this, may I remind you that some of the words that will come out of your mouth will be "forgive us our trespasses, as we forgive those, who trespass against us." In other words, "forgive me to the same degree with which I forgive others," there is no statement in there that says "forgive me because I didn't mean to do it, but they did, so they don't count."

Why would this be in The Lord's Prayer? Because forgiveness is essential, in a civilised society, for our emotional growth and wellbeing.

Forgive them. For your sake forgive them.

Write down a few names or incidents that have happened that you find it difficult to get over – I suspect it may be time to let go.

Action ...

Revisit these from time to time over the next few days and work on forgiveness. Keep working on it, because occasionally they can pop up again and need to be put back into the forgiven box once more.

30

It's Not the Fact

☦

Facts are funny things aren't they? To one person one fact can mean one thing and to another it means something completely different. For example, in Britain we go on about the weather – it rains too frequently and the sun doesn't shine often enough. I have just returned from Australia where the farmers are experiencing a 5 year drought and are desperate for water. If you ask most of the people who have emigrated to Oz, about why they went, there will usually be something in their answer that relates to the weather.

Let's look at another example - If you like watching any team sport, imagine your team are winning the game until 1 minute before the end when the other team score, the game ends as a draw. Most of your team's supporters will go home disappointed, spending a disproportionate amount of time talking about the last minute, but if you had been supporting the other team and in the last minute your team had turned the tables, you would be going home elated.

I once heard a terrific story about an insurance salesman (and I heard this one from the salesman himself so I have no reason to doubt its validity). The salesman was looking after a large client who had a car dealership in Florida. The car dealership was massive; they had just built a new showroom, the fanciest showroom you can imagine. Our salesman went down to the grand opening of the new showroom, (it was a fancy affair with the local Mayor and various dignitaries in attendance) and having checked all insurances were up to date, the salesman returns to his offices in another state.

A couple of months later a hurricane hit Florida with the majority of its force focussed on the town in which the dealership was situated. After hearing of the disaster, the salesman rang the owner to ask what could be done, only to be told that the new showroom was completely destroyed. However, all the staff had had a meeting and decided that while they had no cars to sell they should spend their time helping the town's residents to clean up, which was exactly what they were doing. The owner was in pretty good spirits considering that his beautiful building had been decimated, his reasoning went something like this …

"Well, once we were actually using the showroom, we started to realise a few mistakes we had made in the design, so this was a great opportunity to put them right."

Also during the cleanup campaign one member of staff had a bright idea of collecting all the dead reptiles which the hurricane had picked up and thrown into the town during the storm. These alligators and snakes were to be stuffed. A month later the business had an Alligator sale, 'buy your replacement car and receive a free stuffed Gator as a souvenir of the hurricane'.

This car dealership did more business in the month following the storm than in any previous month in its history. I wonder what the other businesses were doing during the days and weeks that followed the storm.

We all experience storms – it isn't these that weaken us it is the way we choose to react to them that matters.

When something negative happens to you during the next week say to yourself – it isn't the fact but how I react to the fact that determines the outcome. Then choose the outcome you would like and thus your reaction. This process in your head will speed up as you get better at it.

Quick Recall Session

- Every thought we have, every single day, makes a difference to our conditioning either negatively or positively
- We can take control of the way we think
- Focus on what you want to achieve – focus on the end goal and then decide <u>how</u> you need to think about it
- After you have decided what your goals are work out the behaviours that are required to achieve that goal
- The past is gone and nothing will change it – what we must do is focus on the present to achieve what we want in the future
- Learn from the past and move on
- Get over it and get on with it
- Learn to forgive and if you can't forgive and forget at least forgive and move on
- Same facts + different attitude = different outcome
- Its your future – you decide

"The most powerful thing you can do to change the world is to change your own beliefs about the nature of life, people and reality to something more positive ... and begin to act accordingly."

Shakti Gawain, Writer.

31

Great Beginnings

✞

What are you like in the mornings? How do you start your day off? I have been known to allow the radio to wake me up which is quite a shock to the system. But I have to admit it is hard to find a DJ who is going to waken you positively. Most have a moan about the morning, the weather, the news, the people around them etc. This morning the weather person told me that the day would be close and uncomfortable, last week they said it would be dull and dreary! Is that a good start to the day? It is usually done in a humorous way and that's supposed to make it OK, but is it good to start our day off with negatives? Maybe we aren't even giving ourselves a chance.

Music may be a good way to start off. Something pleasant, something that puts a smile on your face, without shocking you into the day. Maybe it would be a good idea to put together a tape of music that starts off gently pleasant and works its way up to a good beat and great lyrics. Obviously this is subjective.

Most people have a routine; it is great to have a routine provided it is a positive one. Instead of reading the bad news in the newspaper first thing maybe there is another way of doing it. There are loads of books published with a positive message in them. Some are like this one with short sessions to read or stories of success. Maybe a book about something you want to learn. I'm not talking about a three hour stint or hard slog, but a 10-20 minute positive zap in the morning. Dance around the kitchen to your favourite record, make your partner stare!!

Get some great thoughts going. When you get in your car, on the bus or off on your journey by foot or train, listen to a great tape; if you are on your own find something great to think about. Become creative; don't think about the same thing for weeks on end, it will lose its impact. Maybe write a quick list of 3 behaviours you are going to concentrate on for that day.

For example you may decide that today is going to be a day of tolerance and that nothing will disturb your peace of mind today.
Just go over it in your mind, what do you want out of today?

Write down here what do you want out of today? (Make it inspiring).

For the next week – when you wake up close your eyes and choose your day, choose your reactions, decide what you will be like that day. Once you have decided, then get up and face the day, make it yours.

Remember this ...

Every Day above Ground Is a Good Day

32

Fantastic Endings

✟

How do you end your day? To be really honest I am better off at starting the day well that I am at ending it well. This doesn't mean my attitude fails me, I'm talking about when I get into bed and I know that it's one of the best times to read something positive, that will bop around in my brain all the time when I am asleep, however, at that time of night I often just want to either crash out or read something light and entertaining.

It takes quite a bit of self discipline. In fact nothing we have talked about has been rocket science, it is all very simple, the key has to be self discipline and that improves the more we do it. It is a bit of a vicious circle; one needs self discipline to do it and doing it will give us self discipline.

Maybe the key is to set ourselves small targets instead of huge targets. The target to read something positive for 10 minutes before one goes to sleep is most likely to be more easily and frequently achieved than the target to read a whole chapter of a book each evening.

Maybe it also helps to set the target short term, for example, being determined to do it every day for 10 days and see how one progresses, can be a great incentive rather than the larger task of, 'I must do this for the rest of my life or I have failed'.

As I said in the introduction I have deliberately set these sessions up to be done three times a week. So that you can either, read the same one a couple of times and really take it in, or think about the content and your interpretation for a couple of days before moving on. Smaller bite size pieces.

On the next page write down some ideas for finishing your day on a positive note (it doesn't have to involve alcohol!).

Maybe you would prefer to vary your endings ...

Monday: 10 minutes reading a personal development book

Tuesday: Play relaxation tape and visualise achieving my goals

Wednesday: Watch a favourite except from a film that gives me feel good factor.

Thursday: Listen to a personal development audio tape or something inspiring

The idea is to combat some of the negatives that hit us during the day and can have a habit of wearing down our good intentions. Don't let them. On the days when we don't feel worn down it is an ideal opportunity to get a head start on tomorrow.

Remember if you leave a garden unattended for a while, it does not remain the same, it grows weeds and our minds are just the same. We need constant attention and work.

Conscious effort to maintain a healthy set of neurological connections.

Go on, you know you can do it.

33

Goals or Dreams

✟

During a survey at Harvard business school, mid way through the 20th Century, I am told that all the students leaving were asked if they had goals. 93% did not have goals; 4% had unwritten goals and 3% had goals written down.

It is said that 20 years later the survey was followed up and the 4% who had unwritten goals had achieved more than the 93% without goals but that the 3% who had written goals, had achieved more and were happier, better adjusted people than all the other 97% put together. Wow, that is quite a survey result.

These results have been used to prove that writing down goals is an essential key to achieving success. In my opinion this is true.

I would like to add another dimension to it. This survey may not necessarily tell us that writing down a goal is the key, what it may tell us, is that people whose behaviours include writing things down in the form of goals are the type of people who will achieve and be better adjusted.

Whichever point it proves to us, we must hold fast to the idea that, some people are born with particular traits and certain natural talents and some develop them. It is never too late and in my opinion very little is impossible.

I have noticed that those who are most successful – and of course it does depend on how you define success – are ones who concentrate on the <u>behaviours</u> it takes to achieve their goals not necessarily the ones who concentrate on the goals.

You see a behaviour can be a lasting trait, but a goal once it is achieved, is often a finite thing. Many people set a goal and once they have achieved it relax back into their previous way of life. How many people do you know who have set a goal to get fit by running a half marathon or full marathon for that matter? Then, once they have run the race, gradually they stop running and return to their 'normal' way of life. Some constantly set goal after goal, but some chose a behaviour and work on 'being' – Lao Tsu said "the way to do is to be."

Behaviour is the 'being' the goal is the 'doing'. Maybe we need both.

Sometimes the behaviour that accompanies a goal can be difficult to define, but if we work on it, we can find it.

Think of the goals you wrote down a few sessions ago. Write them down here again …

In your opinion, what behavioural traits do people who have achieved that sort of goal have?

Which ones do you need to work on?

Focus on these behavioural traits and the thought processes that go along with them over the next few days.

34

Insanity

✟

There are many definitions of insanity – the one I like best (not including the humorous ones) goes like this –

"Insanity is doing the same thing over and over again and expecting a different result." By this definition are we not <u>all</u> insane?

Our dislike of change causes us to continue doing the same thing over and over again and if someone comes along and changes things we complain – even if we didn't like doing it in the first place.

As a parent I know this only too well, I catch myself saying the same things, over and over again and wondering why they aren't having more of an effect.

Maybe it's time to do something different!

People tell me that they want to get more out of their staff at work. They have used the usual motivational tools – threats of job cuts, appraisals, pointing out what they are doing wrong and stamping around, slamming doors, looking miserable and angry.

Maybe it's time to do something different!

Many ladies and gentlemen who wish to lose weight, tell me of the many diets they have tried that don't work, where they cut out this and that and starve themselves until they feel miserable.

Maybe it's time to do something different!

No matter what the problem is, I can usually guarantee that when someone comes up with a new way of tackling it, there are a hundred excuses as to why it won't work for them.

Why?

Breaking the Mirror

Because we have an aversion to change, "just in case" – I wonder what we are so afraid of. It may not work! That's right, it may not work but then the thing we are currently doing isn't working either, so what have we got to lose? Effort, energy, disappointment, maybe we'll learn something new, and discover something revolutionary.

Go on - try doing something different – Fed up of traffic jams? – Try bus, train or bike. Tired of shouting at the kids? – Try talking calmly and persistently – Irritated by constantly forcing yourself to diet? – Try increasing your exercise instead. (I know there are many other ways).

Do something different.

Heather Wright

35

The Luckiest Person in the World

✠

I was cornered by a rather drunk lady one night after I had delivered an after dinner speech to a group. Her opening line was "That was a great speech…" which personally I think is a good opening gambit … but it sort of went down hill from there as she followed it with, "but do you really believe all that stuff about being positive?" Unfortunately, I didn't get a chance to answer before she launched into various things that had happened to her which were, in her opinion, just 'plain lucky'.

Some people are just are lucky then. Aren't they? And some just aren't. To some people, life is a series of co-incidences, being in the right place at the right time. You can't deny it; it's useful if you happen to know someone, who knows someone else, who owns a company, with a vacancy that just suits you. What about the lucky person who co-incidentally bumps into a person with exactly the expertise they were looking for? Wow, that was lucky.

Or is it? The more I watch people's behaviour the more I am convinced that you make your own luck. This lady talked of 'falling into a job', but would she have been offered a job she hadn't applied for, if she didn't have particular characteristics? Would she have taken a completely new turn in her career if she didn't have the confidence to pull it off (whether scared or not)? There must have been a series of events that led up to the job offer, a series of events that she must have had some influence over.

If we believe ourselves to be unlucky, when an opportunity comes along to change or more forward, we can find a million reasons why we cannot go for it. We may also wipe that incident from our memories, so that we do not see it as a missed opportunity, merely a conversation with a colleague.

I heard of a golfer (and this story has been attributed to different ones at different times, so I will not put a name to it) who, when told he was lucky, retorted "yes I am, and the more I practise, the luckier I get."

We have to work on our luck, we have to seize situations and turn them to our advantage; we have to explore passing conversations a little deeper before we decide whether to put them into the recycle bin of our mind.

I have been told that we are all supposed to be six people away from anyone in the world. For example I know a lady, who knows Richard Branson, who knows the Prime Minister. So I am three people away from the Prime Minister! Therefore anyone who knows me is four people away from him, that's if they don't have a closer contact themselves.

Does that mean that there is always a way to get to know people, who may know people, who need our talents. I guess it depends on whether you are a lucky person or not!

On the next page write down all of the lucky things that have happened to you that you can remember.

What about all the co-incidences?

Also all the people you know, who know someone, who could be important to you.

Think lucky; be lucky; remember there *is* a formula to being lucky.

Quick Recall Session

- Start the day off in a fantastic state of mind and you have a greater chance of having a fantastic day
- Choose how the day will go before you react to the events that are put in your path
- Finish the day well and get over as many of today's "facts" as you can – no point in carrying them around with you
- Complete the day on a positive note and it will give you a better chance of starting tomorrow well
- Set specific targets; goals are just written dreams
- Goals can be anything you like – small, medium or big, it's up to you
- If you do what you've always done you'll get what you've always got
- Don't be afraid to be different
- Become a lucky person
- Luck is a formula and a state of mind – it's a choice

A Philosophy on Life

One day several friends were discussing their thoughts about life. They each quoted the saying that meant the most to them.

When it came to the last man, the one who was known for his wisdom, he thoughts for a moment and then quoted his favourite saying from the Bible "And it came to pass."

The others were surprised that he had not chosen a more famous saying, but in answer to their questions he replied:

"This is what I try to remember, sometimes I get so caught up in the past that I forget that things come and go, and that we've got to find the faith to keep going. That phrase is like a window that shows me there's life beyond my momentary problems, even though they feel like a prison. It helps me keep my head up and my spirit strong – there's a path out there and it's my job to find it."

Adapted from - "A Complete Treasury of Stories for Public Speakers."

36

What Drives You?

✟

If we teach people to say "Have a nice day" to everyone they meet, some will say it with great feeling, make all their contacts feel great and talk about what a wonderfully caring person they have just met. However, some will say the same words but the tone, body language and implication behind the words, will turn it into an aggressive, patronizing or purely robotized statement. The difference is, as many people have said before me, not what you say but how you say it.

How you say it comes from your motivation for saying it. I.e. "I will say have a nice day because I have been told to, even though I don't give a ha'penny about whether you drop down dead as soon as you are round the corner, so long as you don't do it in front of me because that would be mightily inconvenient," is a different motivation to, "I am a great person and I have no doubt you are and I know that by saying this to you it may well pass on a small piece of positive feeling and therefore make a difference to you."

This motivation comes from the core of one's being – our driving force. Our set of values, we may even call this our 'raison d'étre'. If our core is right then the strategy will be right, but if the core is wrong, then we can employ many different strategies and they will not make that difference.

In the past when I have recommended to others that a particular course of action could start with the words, "I'm sorry" the response can often be, "why should I say sorry, I've done nothing wrong?!" What is the problem with saying sorry? If by saying sorry the emphasis shifts from trying to determine blame to, getting to a point where positive action can be taken, then it is surely the right thing to do. In my opinion, we can often be far too caught up in our need to maintain our status, ie "If I say sorry, they will thing I am in the wrong" or "backing down" or "weak" etc. however, if by saying sorry the other person can be refocused onto the important issue, then surely the rest does not matter. Maybe it stems from our

Breaking the Mirror

increasingly litigious society? But I fear the battle for status lies far deeper and is far older than that.

When teaching conflict management one of the key points is to decide the desired outcome of the conflict and work towards it without getting caught up in side issues of power and emotion.

This is a tough one, and takes a great deal of self awareness. You may be someone who hasn't given it much thought or you maybe extremely self aware.

Over the next few days spend a little extra time exploring which emotions drive the things you say. Ask yourself – "why did I say that, what was my motivation?"

37

Core and Strategy

✞

Imagine this

You are single and at a party, you begin to talk to someone to whom you are attracted, not only in looks, but also in personality. You find that you have much in common, liking the same kind of movies, books, sports etc. You decide to meet again. On the first date you are both early, flowers are given and received, chocolates are bought and eaten and an effort is made with regard to appearance. The relationship continues until you know each other very well and decide to spend the rest of your lives together.

The time you have spent together so far has been building a core or a foundation. The compliments you have exchanged, both verbally and in action, have said to each other that you love one another.

The desire to impress by turning up on time, bringing unsolicited gifts, wearing clothes that the other will find attractive says to that person – You are important to me, what you think and do matters.

This is part of your combined core.

Outside of this core is a strategy, the strategy gets you to where you are going. This core in any relationship must be built very strongly in order for the relationship to endure any set backs. The strategy is how we get to where we wish to be, which in the case of the scenario above, is a happy long term relationship.

For instance getting married or living together is a strategy, many people have married without the core in place and it has not lasted, but the opposite is also true. Some people say that they have a good laugh with their partner and that includes negative banter and negative humour.

This only works provided the core is firmly in place and is also maintained. For example provided the core is in place, those comments like, "I wish you wouldn't pick your feet in bed" or "I only married you so that you would do the ironing and make the bed," can be taken in good humour without causing distress. These comments are usually just about strategy, for example, "life would be more pleasant if you didn't pick your feet in bed" or "… leave your clothes on the bathroom floor" but they can cause one person to "go home to mothers!!" All because the core is or is not in place.

The core, once in place, needs maintenance (just like a house needs rendering or painting) or one day you wake up and find that it is in a dreadful state and one little negative destroys the whole thing.

If the relationship breaks down at this point, the post mortem is unlikely to be "you asked me not to pick my feet in bed, so I can't live with you any more," it is more often that one was, "taken for granted" or "constantly criticism" or it's that we "never talk anymore."

The same is true with friendships, before we can use any negatives with another individual, we must have built and maintained a firm core.

I made this mistake a little while ago, when a friend asked for my 'honest' opinion and I gave it, warts and all. Oops. I had thought that we had a solid core in place and it would not do any harm, however, my comments smouldered for 6 months before I took my friend to one side and said "what's wrong?" – The reply was along the lines of "you told me I was an awful person." Actually my perception was that I said "I think you are a wonderful person and we all have faults but I love you anyway and although I have noticed this fault it has not stopped me liking you."

If our core had been in place as firmly as I had thought it was, my comments which were only strategic, would have been taken on at that level and not on a deeper level.

Luckily we were able to have that conversation; I was able to clarify my unfortunate and less than diplomatic approach and I have spent much time since then, repairing the breach in our relationship.

Those people we have a good core built up with are the ones we can take a little negative strategy from – who can you handle honesty from?

Try the exercise on the next page.

Put the people who you have most contact with or are most important in your life into three categories

Solid Core

Some core

No core.

Think about each person you meet and consider your relationship with them – we will use these thoughts during the rest of the book.

38

Solid Relationships

✞

This core and strategy model applies to many instances, when looking at company values and mission statements, when looking at managing staff, looking at personal relationships and at our own behaviour and driving force.

There are only so many people one can build a solid core with on a deeper level. For instance some management books may say that no-one can 'manage' more than 10 people. Whether 10 is the correct figure or not is irrelevant to us at this stage; each company/person must decide for themselves. The point is this – in order for us to 'manage' someone effectively we must build a solid relationship and that takes time, effort and thought. Time is the one limitation we can never change, there will always be 24 hours in the day and 7 days to a week (and if you are reading this book in the year 4389 and this is no longer true, it is time for a reprint!). We may fit more activities into each day but people are different.

Therefore there will be a limit to how many people we can personally build that relationship with. This figure will depend upon the type of person you are and the type of person your 'friend' is. Some people are better at 'building' than others, two of such types will reach a level of understanding far quicker than one of these types and for someone who is less able/willing, 'building' that core will take even longer especially when both personality types find relationships challenging to say the least.

This of course also applies in our personal lives. We have different levels of friends. In its simplest terms, there are surface level acquaintances, someone you have a chat with, maybe someone you have a laugh with but wouldn't want to share your deep personal problems with. Then there are friends who you see frequently, therefore know more about and talk about how you feel with and then there are those, who you consider to be extended family (please note the I am using the word family here to depict a depth of friendship rather than whether or not one is related to them). Some of these friends or extended family have such a firmly built up 'core' that it sometimes doesn't take a lot to maintain. But these are the people you may call when you really need a friend.

Relatives can be similar to friends in that a core built up firmly during childhood can mean that frequent contact is not always necessary. But one cannot assume that purely because one spent a childhood with a relative that a core was actually built. The amount of people we all meet who have massive chips on their shoulders because of relatives can be quite shocking, but often when we look beyond that initial gripe, there can still be a solid core built up. Maybe the line from the song, *'Affirmation'* by Savage Garden sums it up, "I believe my parents did the best job they knew how to do." Maybe, although we may moan about our relatives, we should understand that we are all novices when it comes down to it.

Anyway back to friends and colleagues: How many of your friends do you think you have a good core friendship with and how many colleagues? What do you consciously do to help build that core up? What else will you do from now on? Write a list of the people who have the most influence on your life and beside their name write down what you do now to build the core between you and some ideas about what else you can do.

Work on building relationships with people, decide which ones it is easier to do so with and with which ones you most desire to do so, also add those who should be on the list because having a good relationship would make life easier. What can you do over the next 7 days or month that will help these relationships?

Write down some people's names below and ideas for building your relationships – base these ideas on where your relationship is now and what type of people they are.

39

Self Talk (1 of 7)

✝

This subject is a very important one so I have written 7 sections on it.

We will be considering our self talk over the next few chapters and working on really getting to grips with it.

Self talk is the conversation we have with ourselves all day, every day, 24/7. Obviously we can't control every little thought from the start, but what we can do, is develop great self talk habits that will eventually lead to our less conscious thoughts being great ones.

First of all I would like to split self talk into three categories. It is not essential to do this but I prefer to do so. The three categories are these ...

    a) generic self talk
    b) specific self talk
    c) triggers or self starters

'Generic self talk' is the supposedly innocent, almost irrelevant, conversation that goes on and manifests itself in face pulling and little moans and groans. For example "Have you seen the weather isn't it horrible? We haven't had much of a summer this year" or "this drink is warm. I don't like tepid water, typical that they don't have any ice, they never get their act together." My opinion is that these things can be an irritation but you can either do something about it or you can let it go.

Moaning becomes a habit with some people and their faces seem to tell us that before they even open their mouths. But remember, every thought we have has an impact on our brains and our bodies, moaning is not the high performance option. I would explain here that I am not suggesting that we don't try to get great service in restaurants and don't try to solve things that have gone wrong, but there is a difference between sorting something out and moaning and complaining. In fact the self talk which says "I am going to complain about this" is not as specific or as helpful as "I am going to get something done about this," one piece of self talk is focussed on moaning and venting ones spleen and the other is working towards a solution. Obviously we may not always get the solution we were looking for but if we set off with the right self talk we will have a better chance of a successful outcome.

Spend some time over the next couple of days becoming aware of the **'generic self talk'** around you. See how much of it is solution orientated and how much is just hot air. Also spend some time noticing how often you do it in your head. The first step is to become aware of it. Then start turning it around so that you are working on a solution rather than focussing on the problem. Don't worry if you don't always come up with a solution, sometimes there isn't one, at those times it is best to focus totally on something else and let it go.

Remember the old adage "If you haven't got anything nice to say don't say anything at all." For some people obeying this would cut out a high proportion of their conversation, but maybe we'd all be better off because of it! I know that I have switched my focus from thought to conversation, but the principle is the same. Please remember that all conversation starts with thought and therefore if we don't think negatively we won't talk negatively. "If you don't have anything nice to think don't think anything at all" may be an extension of the saying, but I would rather change it to "If you don't have anything nice to think … shame on you!"

'Generic self talk' is reactive and takes practice. But if we become aware of it on a daily basis our reactions will become more and more focussed on a positive result.

40

Specific Self Talk (2 of 7)

✟

The next category of self talk is **'specific self talk'**. By this I am talking about the bigger stuff. The things in our lives that, if we could change our behaviour in some way, would be a big deal to us and may make a huge impact on our lives. For example you may have a fear of doing presentations (after all research tells us that giving a presentation is the thing that most people are afraid of in the western world) and you may have a presentation to do in front of your boss or an important client. Or, you may have a particular person you have clashes with on a regular basis and you don't feel comfortable around, it may affect you in a negative way.

It doesn't surprise me that people have a fear of presentations, when you listen to what they say about them, it's enough to scare anybody. Find someone who doesn't like doing them and ask them about presentations. They will invariably say things like "I am scared that I will forget what I am going to say, or that I will make a fool of myself. What if I can't answer any questions or they laugh at me? I might fall over and look a complete idiot." Well, with that comforting picture in my head I think I would be pretty scared too.

I was once at an exam, waiting along with the others who were due to take it, the atmosphere was tense and people were rushing back and forth to the toilet and outside for nervous cigarettes. A family of four were standing around, two adults and two children aged below 14, they talked of the things they were most nervous about, they talked about the mistakes they had made when they were practising and built up a horror film of potential disasters in their heads together, they were very creative. By the time the youngest child went in to the room he was a bundle of nerves and it didn't surprise me to hear that as soon as the examination started he burst in to tears.

In order to get our **'specific self talk'** right we need to start with the performance we require and work backwards.

What is the performance you would love to have?

Now make it a brighter picture, what is the performance you would really love to have?

For example "I'd like to get through the presentation without making a fool of myself" is not a particularly exciting thought is it? But the idea of running the presentation in a professional, smooth and polished manner, slotting in extra information where appropriate, elaborating on points when required and the boss coming up to you afterwards, patting you on the back and saying well done you were terrific; now that's a picture that makes you excited.

Find a powerful picture, one of confidence and success, however you would define it.

Then ask yourself what sort of self talk you need to give a performance like that.

Maybe put it into the third person if you are struggling, who do you know whose performance would be the sort you would like, what do you think their self talk is.

Then adapt it to fit yourself.

Heather Wright

Write down specific behaviours or performances that you would like to change …

Now write down your current self talk about them …

Breaking the Mirror

Now write down the behaviours or performances you would prefer (remember make them powerful) …

Now write down the self talk you would need in each case in order to get that particular behaviour or performance...

Think about it, and keep coming back to it over the next day or so.

Quick Recall Session

- Motivation does not come from the strategy we employ – i.e. wearing bright clothes, saying have a nice day – it comes from within
- What is our driving force; our reason for being; our personal vision?
- Relationships on all levels are based on how securely our core is built
- The core needs maintenance
- We must work at building a solid core with the people who have an influence on our lives
- We can only have difficult or negative conversations with others once we have build a solid core
- Self talk is every little thought we have, every minute of the day
- Self talk can be positive, neutral or negative
- We need to develop positive self talk to overcome our negatives

*"Things do not happen.
They are made to happen."*

John F. Kennedy,
(1917–1963),
35th U.S. President

41

Self Talk – Triggers (3 of 7)

✞

The third category of self talk is **'self starters or triggers'**. These are usually used as either an intervention or a booster. In other words if you are having trouble with negative self talk these are a fast track to getting yourself on a more positive path. Long drawn out self talk may not be the answer for you. It may be possible for you to get the results you want by using a short phrase which brings up a picture of the end result you want.

Mohammed Ali had many different triggers, some were specific to a particular fight but some were general ones, "I am the greatest" was general and no doubt boosted his self belief every time he said it. Tommy Steele the entertainer is known to have said "I'm home" before he walked onto the stage. The trigger to feeling more relaxed and comfortable in what must sometimes be a frightening place.

Liverpool Football Club have the phrase "THIS IS ANFIELD" on a sign above the tunnel leading to the pitch (which the team then reach up and touch as they walk into their stadium). Imagine the effect this would have on any footballer, but especially on some young man, who has dreamed of playing football for a premier league side all his life. Imagine the negative effect on a team, with a belief that they are already the under-dogs, when they see the sign.

Many people have negative triggers which work very well and encourage them to feel bad. Do you recognise any of the following?

"The bubble's bound to burst"

"Why me"

"It always happens to me"

"I'm so unlucky"

"I hate Mondays"

There are some great triggers, but it is essential you use one that brings up the right picture for you, try these for size or invent your own …

"Simply the best"

"Go for it"

"You're better than that"

"Get over it"

"I feel terrific"

"I'm on a roll"

"Come on"

All of these can be negative triggers if the feeling behind them isn't right, only you will know what pictures and thus feelings they generate in you, which is why it is not a great idea for me to give you too many examples.

Remember it's not the words alone but your tone of voice and body language that adds to the power of a trigger and thus the picture drawn in your head.

Over the next few days develop a few triggers that work for you. They can be used to refocus yourself, to raise your mood, to celebrate a success or anything you need. It could be lines from an inspiring film or something that reminds you of an event in your past. Whatever works for you.

Write down your first thoughts below and give them a try over the next few days ...

42

Self Talk (4 of 7)

✠

Self talk is the conversation you have with yourself all day every day. Every little thought, significant or not, is part of your self talk. These thoughts build up a picture of yourself and your world.

There is a full blown commentary going on in your head right now. A lot of it is filed away, before you consciously realise you have thought it, but it still goes on. You walk into a room and you think about the temperature, the atmosphere, the cleanliness, the positions of the furniture, the colour of the walls, how you feel about the whole thing and so on.

Breaking the Mirror

One of the first things to remember is that every thought you have, and I mean EVERY ONE creates a physical link in the brain, either by travelling down and thus reinforcing an existing one or creating a new one. Thoughts aren't just your conscious thoughts they include expressions and are linked to your body language and vocal tone.

It is no use trying to cheat by figuring that you can think in a certain way during a particular activity i.e. whilst playing golf or squash and then think in a different way later on when going over the game in your head or with a friend. The sports people I have worked with have often been the most difficult to convince of this fact. It does make a difference. So we can't just say one thing to the coach and then quietly go off and think something else; it will affect you. Obviously when you start thinking differently, it can be quite a challenge, especially if you have been a negative thinker or maybe a worrier for many years. You will have a thoroughly worn pathway in your head and therefore, purely by the fact that repetition of a thought increases the likelihood of further repetition, you may have created quite a challenging habit.

Good news, there are ways however, to make changing this habit (thought pattern) easier and no matter how long you have been thinking one way, I believe it is possible to change. But my first question to you is, "how much do you want to change?" Without the desire to change your way of thinking there will be many excuses we can come up with for why we 'cannot' rather than 'don't want to'.

Remember: if you do what you've always done you will get what you've always got.

Maybe it is time for a few changes. It is up to you. Some people don't want to admit that they should change because they worry that they will fail, and for those people trying to do something and then failing, is worse than not trying in the first place.

Ask yourself – how do I feel about changing the way I think? If I knew for a fact that I could achieve what I really want to be, by changing the way I think, would I want to? Is it fear of failure that holds me back? Is it lack of belief in my ability to change? Or am I ready to make a serious go of it?

Become aware of your self talk and notice how many of your thoughts are negative and therefore unhelpful to your goals and dreams. Try to filter out some of the negative ones and turn them into positive ones.

There will be more about how to do this over the next sessions so don't worry if you don't get it right straight away.

43

Self Talk 5 of 7

✟

Our thoughts are not in words. We think in pictures. Young children who do not understand their language yet are still able to think. Words are what we to use to build the pictures in our head.

For instance the word dog brings up a different picture for everyone but the word Terrier makes it more defined. However, we still don't have a particularly good picture, so it would be better to add some descriptive words. "The happy, yappy, fuzzy little terrier was the delight of the blond haired bubbly enthusiastic 6 year old boy who had wanted a puppy since he was very small. He loved to chase sticks and often played games with the children in his street." The picture is starting to become clearer.

An important point to make at this juncture is that pictures are always positive. When I use the word positive I do not mean it in its emotional sense, what I mean is that pictures are always "of" something, in other words when we bring up a picture in our head it is a definite picture. Look at a picture somewhere near to you right now. Describe it to yourself in your head.

Okay, now I will bet that you didn't say to yourself, "that picture is of someone not doing ..." nor will you have said "that picture is not of a ....." Pictures are always 'of' something, does that make sense? So when we say to our friend when we are out bowling "whatever you do don't let it go down the gully" the picture in everyone's head is of the bowl going down the gully. When we say to a child "don't step in the puddle" the picture in our heads is of someone stepping in the puddle. We have said over and over that our behaviour is the manifestation of the picture we hold in our head. Therefore, when we tell a child not to step in the puddle, we are drawing a picture in that child's head of 'stepping in the puddle'. This means that they are drawn towards the action of stepping in the puddle and find it difficult not to do so.

If the picture is one with a negative emotion attached to it the incentive may be huge. For example, "if you step in

Breaking the Mirror

the puddle and get your socks and shoes wet I will cancel your birthday party and you will go to bed early everyday for a week," may be enough of a negative picture to prevent the occurrence, but then the picture has moved from stepping in the puddle to an unhappy child with no birthday party. However, it should not be necessary to negatively motivate someone, if the picture we draw in their head is a better one. For example "Walk around the edge of the puddle and keep yourself perfectly dry"

Write the positive pictures to these commonly heard phrases …

"Whatever you do don't miss the goal"

"Don't run in the corridors"

"Don't talk with your mouth full"

Heather Wright

"Don't look now"

"Don't forget to pick up the dry cleaning"

Now go through them again and make the picture even brighter by adding descriptive positive words.

"I love it when we walk round the puddle and keep our clothes pristine – it makes me really proud"

Notice how many negative instructions people around you give today and mentally swap them round. It can sometimes be quite hard, but it gets easier with practice.

44

Self Talk (6 of 7)

✝

Now we have a better idea of drawing positive pictures for ourselves in our self talk we can spend some time on the language we use.

Remember that words draw pictures in our head which release emotions into our system. I would like to spend some time now looking at the words we use when we are drawing the pictures.

It important to remember what we said earlier about our frame of reference, words don't have meaning; it is people that give them meaning. I would like to add to that and say that 'tone of voice and body language also make a huge difference'. Obviously one person can use what may usually sound negative and make it sound wonderful and obviously the opposite is also true.

But for now let's concentrate on the words. There is no hard and fast rule over these so I am not going give a definitive list of negative words and positive words; I am going to use a few generic examples. For example the word problem has a negative reflex within us. Imagine your boss or partner ringing you and saying "I need to see you immediately we have a problem" – that would give us a terrible feeling wouldn't it, even before we know what the problem actually is. If we are unable to see that person immediately to find out what it is all about, we may imagine all sorts of terrible things that could possibly have gone wrong and by the time we are face to face we have gone through all sorts or hell.

Some people have suggested changing the word 'problem' to the word 'opportunity' and when it was first done and I can imagine that being quite successful. However I have come across a lot of cynicism over that one recently and so now we have a sense of negativity over the problem and also a sense that we are having the wool pulled over our eyes as well. I have also used the word 'challenge', in the past, and that has often worked for me, but unfortunately it can often be tarred with the same brush as 'opportunity'.

What we need to do is focus forwards on what needs to be done instead of the 'problem'. Maybe it would be possible to say "we need a solution for something and, as you are the most creative one I know, would you come and see me so that we can throw some ideas around". Obviously this is not a definitive answer; you may need to get some more urgency into it but what we don't want to do, is start people worrying and thus seize up the brain and its creativity. Fear and worry are great at curbing all our ideas.

Another example is the word 'but'. It is such a little innocuous word and yet it negates everything that has gone before it. If what has gone before it is negative then 'but' can be useful and there are times when it is necessary. Many times it is slipped into a sentence without really thinking about it, maybe just to join one part of a sentence to another and then the damage is done. 'However' is not a suitable alternative, so my suggestion (and it is just a suggestion) is the word 'and'. Sometimes the two words interchange readily and other times there is a need to change the whole structure of the sentence. However you do it and whatever word you pick, it is important to remember that once something has been said, it cannot be unsaid. So we need to pick our words carefully.

Heather Wright

Notice the words people use and how they enhance or detract from the picture that they are drawing in our heads. Write a list of words that have negative connotations for you and then try and find some better replacements ...

45

Self Talk (7 of 7)

✟

Our self talk builds our picture of who we are in our head. This becomes our self concept. Our self concept then becomes so deeply ingrained it is how we explain our behaviour to ourselves or others. For example, "I'm always doing that, I'm so clumsy," is a self concept. This self concept shows itself in our beliefs and expectations. When our self concept is etched into our minds we start to have expectations of how we will behave or perform even when thinking about the things we have never done before. I know many people who believe they will be no good at skiing even before they have tried it. Before most of us set foot in the bowling alley we have an expectation as to what sort of score we will get.

In the long term we perform exactly as we expected to. Our performance then fuels our self talk but not necessarily according to our performance, oh no, it fuels it accordingly to our already built self concept or self image. For example we have all heard of those who have a great expectation and then blame their tools when their performance is not up to scratch, or the person with a low expectation apologise to those around them for performing well claming it to be a "fluke" or "beginner's luck." Then, of course, our self talk enhances our self concept and our performance follows.

Many times people struggle to change their performance without changing their self concept first. It is essential to change our self talk then the rest will follow. Our obsession with being right must not interfere with great self talk.

It never bothered Muhammad Ali when he started telling himself at an early age that he was "the greatest." He started that wonderful piece of self talk when he was still at school and yet surely there is no way that a young boy could be "the greatest." But eventually his performance, driven by a great deal of hard work, fulfilled his self talk. One of the amazing things I love about Muhammad Ali is that his self talk also influenced his opponents. Maybe he was one of the first sports psychologists. Muhammad Ali regularly told his opponent in which round they go down in and in 17 out of 19 fights he got it right. When Ali said "Archie Moore down in four" often enough, it would ring in his opponents ears, then of course when the bell goes and it is announced "round four" what was Archie Moore thinking about?

Great self talk builds a fantastic self concept and a brilliant performance follows. Ask yourself what your self talk needs to be in order to achieve your goals. I bet you don't feel the need to achieve your goals by thinking about all your mistakes and how lousy you are. Write some examples of your current self concept down (It's OK – it's just between you and me).

Quick Recall Session

- Our thoughts are in pictures
- The words we use build those pictures
- We need to build positive pictures to inspire us to positive action
- Be careful of the words you use – they are important
- Our self concept is our strongest motivator – i.e. "I did that because I am that kind of a person"
- To change our behaviour permanently we must use our thoughts/self talk to change our self concept
- Short triggers are a quick and effective way to make instant changes
- Develop some great triggers to drive you through some of your usual barriers and out the other side
- Develop positive self talk habits which will become real physical pathways in the brain and thus affect our behaviour and, of course, our further self talk

"One ought every day at least, to hear a little song, read a good poem, see a fine picture, and, if it were possible, to speak a few reasonable words."

Johann Wolfgang Von Goethe, (1749–1832), Writer

46

Words

✝

We put so much importance on words now-a-days and yet we spend so little time thinking before we speak. Words that have been said can never be un-said; it's like trying to get toothpaste back into the tube. I find as I think back over my life that I have often regretted speaking hastily but I have rarely regretted choosing to say nothing.

We speak in the heat of the moment and cause untold damage to the recipient of our thoughtless words. Sometimes we don't even perceive that what we have said is hurtful but what is received has been barbed and cutting.

I wonder how often I have walked away from a conversation with someone not knowing that they have perceived my words in such a way that they are hurt or angry.

Obviously we cannot always blame ourselves for the perceptions of others, as it may be something totally out of our control, maybe they have an old wound which we have unintentionally touched upon. But I wonder if we could make a difference to the percentage of misunderstandings caused by poorly chosen words that express more than we originally intended.

I once read a book about communication and the author explained that as we grow up we are taught to speak to show how much we know. For example, at school the questions are fired at us and we raise our hand in the hope of receiving some satisfaction or even praise, because we knew the answer. That may never leave us. There is a desire to prove to others how much we know. I have noticed in a training environment, how often I ask delegates to look at a particular puzzle and yet not tell anyone else what they see, so that they do not spoil it for the others and to let them find the answer in their own time. Yet some still feel the need to and at the very least place their paper loudly down, with a noise of some sort, to let everyone know that they have found the answer. It surprises me even more how many of these adults cannot resist saying the answer out loud. Thus saying to the world "I know the answer," letting everyone know how clever they are.

When I considered this in my own conversation, I noticed the same need to let others know how much I knew. Obviously when running a seminar or training course this is the point, however, this carried on with subjects that I wasn't teaching or in a social setting. So I started to consider one question before opening my mouth …

"Am I saying this to prove how much I know or am I saying this because it would be helpful to those listening?" I found it changed the content, quantity and hopefully the quality of my words.

47

Drawing Pictures

✟

Still on the subject of words it is important to realise that words mean nothing. We give them meaning, according to our frame of reference. For example a toddler who has never experienced a burn will not fully understand the words of an anxious parent saying, "don't touch the cooker it's hot and will burn you," except that they may understand the tone of voice with which it is being said and have a deeper understanding of the fear they instinctively pick up. But it is not until they have an experience of some kind, which they can attach to it, that they will truly understand what is being said to them.

A friend of mine once asked me to go to the theatre with them. "What's on?" I said "Macbeth," she replied "with Sean Bean." "Hmm ... I like Macbeth but I'm not a big fan of Sean Bean," "not a fan of Sean Bean?" she said incredulously "really!?" "Yes" I replied "he always looks to me like he has bad breath," (apologies to Sean Bean - I'm sure his dental hygiene is perfect) she laughed at me and said we would find something else to go and see. Now why would I think that about someone I have never met (and now I hope will never meet, because it will be just my luck that someone will have told him what I said about his breath!). It's all about frame of reference, in my head the way he looks is attached to a thought about having bad breath. There is no logic in it, but then that's the way it is with someone's frame of reference. We don't have to explore their deep inner meanings, but we do have to acknowledge their existence and thus choose our words carefully.

The words we use draw a picture in our heads and that picture communicates to us, because of our frame of reference. Great authors have amazing skill at using this fact to their advantage. They spend pages using their words to illustrate the surroundings they wish us to see in our minds eye, they describe the feelings of the characters in their story and the situation they have found themselves in. We create images in our minds which bring the book to life, helping us to experience with the characters their emotions. Maybe that is why when Joyce

Grenfell was asked which she preferred TV or Radio she replied, "I prefer the radio. The pictures are much better than on the TV."

When we communicate, we need to choose our words so that they draw a picture in the heads of the recipients, that picture is the thing that communicates our message. I heard a parent telling a child who had to speak on stage recently "don't worry sweet heart, I know how scary it is, but if you forget your words I will prompt you." On the surface that may seem reassuring, but I can't help feeling that the child went on stage with the picture of something really scary in its head and of course the picture of forgetting the lines is not exactly reassuring. Maybe a statement like "Wow sweetheart this is so exciting, when people see you on that stage they are going to think how brilliant and clever you are. I will be so proud sitting close by for any support you need." Obviously there is no definitive answer we just need to think carefully about the consequences of our words.

48

Those Harder Days

✝

Sometimes it just seems impossible doesn't it? The forces of darkness are against you and you don't have the power or strength to fight the fight and win. So you may as well give in. NO! NO! NO!

It's true, some days, weeks or maybe even months seem harder than the other ones, but those are the ones we have to battle with. That is the resistance training that makes you really strong.

COME ON – put on a piece of upbeat music and convince yourself you can handle anything 'they' throw at you. It's the only way – the alternative is untenable.

Life is too short – so they say – and they are right. Be brave, be bold and be determined to fulfil your potential – whatever it is. No-one ever did it by feeling sorry for themselves or indeed worrying about things that will never happen. Besides worrying about things just extends the agony.

Get out a piece of paper and write down ten ways to solve your problems or ten ways to get to where your going – no idea is too strange, no idea is too wacky. (May I suggest keeping within the law!!) Ask yourself "what if?" or "how can I?" It's better to ask questions than to run through negatives in your head.

You never know until you try, you never fail until you stop trying. Take a leaf out of Helen Keller's book – she said "Life is either a daring adventure or nothing" – not bad for someone blind and deaf.

If you are anything like me, there are times when you don't consciously choose to get upset about things but emotions just take over.

Sometimes it's over really big stuff and sometimes it's over piddly little stuff. Whatever the 'stuff' our main problem is not the 'stuff' but the chemicals that flood our systems and make us feel that there is 'no way out' or 'nothing we can do'.

So the first thing to do is to get our body back onto an even keel (chemistry wise) – pick a couple of songs that always make you feel like a million dollars. Depends on what they remind you of. Then play them and sing along loudly. *"Gold … always believe in your soul, you're indestructible, always believe"* etc that's it really go for it!

Flood your system with positive chemicals; it may take a bit longer. Once you have your system more balanced, you may be able to think more clearly or at least give yourself a break.

Go on you deserve it – give yourself a break. Tina Turner *"Simply the Best,"* or *"Don't stop me now"* by Queen.

Maybe you could put on your favourite feel good factor film to change your mood or you could try one of my favourite tactics – I listen to tapes of comedy for example Victoria Wood, Eddie Izzard or Billy Connelly.

On the next page write down all the things that make you laugh or feel good …

Music ...

Comedy people ...

Feel good films ...

Heather Wright

49

Topping Ourselves Up

✟

Have you ever noticed that most of the things we do to cheer ourselves up or to give ourselves that 'feel-good-factor' don't last?

My washing machine broke. It was ten years old, which isn't bad for a washing machine and we decided that it wasn't worth getting it repaired, so we went out to buy a new one. That was quite fun, in a "how many different settings can one family use" kind of way, but having it delivered had a kind of exciting anticipation to it. Delivery between 1 and 5 o'clock we were told, so I waited in, rushing to the window every time any large vehicle went past for 3 hours until the van arrived. A pleasant man with a trolley deposited the new one and took the old one away. It is now sitting with its wrapping and polystyrene still on waiting to be plumbed in and the excitement is already starting to wear off. One or two washes, wondering whether we have chosen the right setting and that will be it.

At that point we need a 'top up'. If we constantly depend on 'having' in order to 'top up' it is a very expensive way of achieving happiness. Surely we need to examine the sorts of thing we do that give us 'feel-good-factor' and why they do that. The only reason for examining why is so that we may be able to add to the list. It may also be a good idea to write a list of the things that detract from our happiness – this list should be written when we are in a positive frame of mind, because if our body is flooded with negative chemicals at the time of writing the list, we may use it to vent our anger, frustration or unhappiness rather than sensibly viewing the matter calmly, in order to work out a plan for placing ourselves in that situation less often.

However, there is a good argument that says if we work on doing more of the things that make us feel good about ourselves, then surely subconsciously we will do less of the stuff that makes us feel bad about ourselves.

So let's start with the positive list, my suggestion would be to start off by just putting down everything that comes into your head whether sensible or even censorable and then sort it out into a usable list.

Make sure you include things that build up your self esteem by working on your values and self concept – for example you may have eating chocolate on your list of things that make you feel good (I know many people would put that down) but what about reading a story to your child or taking a meal round to the elderly friend down the road. Eating the chocolate is purely a feel good event but the other two things are about making you feel good about yourself. Things that make you feel worthy and deserving are important.

'Feel-good-factors'

'Happiness Detractors'

50

The Winning Way

✟

A little boy and girl wanted to meet the wisest man in the world. When they found him, they said, "Sir, we understand that you are one of the wisest men in the world. We want to be like you when we grow up. How can we do that?"

The man responded with these words of wisdom: "Children, there are four words I would like to say to you. When you grow up, you will be very wise if you remember these words and live by them.

"The first word is 'Think'. Think about the values and principles that are important to you."

"The second word is 'Believe'. Believe in yourself based on the thinking you have done."

"The third word is 'Dream'. Dream about what you want to become based on your belief in yourself."

"The last word is 'Dare'. Dare to make your dream a reality."

Then in front of Sleeping Beauty's castle and by Snow White's wishing well, Walt Disney said to the boy and girl

"Let me say those four words again so you can remember them: Think, Believe, Dream and Dare."

What a great story. I don't know if is true but it doesn't really matter. Disney led a life of mixed blessings (actually he led a difficult life by anyone's standards). He tried many different enterprises and failed. He tried some that worked and then something beyond his control let him down.

He borrowed money and lost it, he had ideas stolen but he never stopped trying. According to *"The Little Big Book of Disney"* Walt was in hospital when he told his brother of his idea for Disney World in Florida and died the next day. His brother came out of retirement to make Walt's dream come true and died shortly after succeeding. But what a legacy he left the world.

All because he persisted. Never giving up.

How much persistence have you got? Dogged determination is the key. Think about your values and principles; believe in yourself for it is those values and principles that make you who you are. Dream about the things you would like to do with your life (its never too late – you don't have to be a young child) and then Dare to make those Dreams a reality. Why not? You have everything to gain, some things take time – getting started is half the battle. Go for it!!

What are you going to do that is different from what you were doing when you started this journal?

What is your vision? Who are you to be?

I believe that God created all people equal, we have special talents and different personalities but, to all He gave the ability to choose, to all He gave access to Him, to all He gave ... and gave ... and gave ...

Our job is to seize the opportunities that we have been given.

Quick Recall Session

- Pay attention to the words that come out of your mouth and how they can be received
- Don't speak just to prove how much you know
- Ask yourself, before you speak – is it the truth? Is it kind? Is it helpful?
- We all have tougher days – its how you handle them that matters
- Use techniques to prevent getting bogged down
- Everyone needs some help to keep up a better attitude
- Develop a simple system to use for when you need a top up
- Seize the opportunities in life
- Learn from the mistakes you make
- Stay on the right path towards your goals

Conclusion

✟

Well we have come to the end of this particular journey together and I sincerely pray that it has been useful to you. Small bits; little things to think about. You may not have agreed with everything I have put down, that doesn't matter, I place my thoughts on the paper to make you think, to question, to analyse things you may otherwise have not considered.

I have not overtly mentioned my faith in the pages of this book, but I hope it has been obvious how important it is. If you do not have a faith or do not believe in God then I trust that you will get just as much from this journal, and maybe, deep down you will find faith because if what I have written is correct and truthful, then all truth is God's truth.

Finally ...

Be grateful – "Gratitude unlocks the fullness of life. It turns what we have into enough and more. It turns denial into acceptance, chaos into order, confusion to clarity. It can turn a meal into a feast, a house into a home, a stranger into a friend. Gratitude makes sense of our past, brings peace for today, and creates vision for tomorrow." (Melody Beatie – Writer).

Be confident – "Delight yourself in the Lord and He will give you the desires of your heart." (Psalm 37:4).

Be humble – "Do nothing from selfishness or empty conceit, but with humility of mind let each of you regard one another as more important than himself; do not merely look out for your own personal interests, but also for the interests of others." (Philippians 2:3-4).

This is a day that the Lord has made – let us rejoice and be glad in it.

"Our deepest fear is not that we are inadequate. Our deepest fear is that we are powerful beyond measure. It is our light, not our darkness, that most frightens us. We ask ourselves, who am I to be brilliant, gorgeous, talented, fabulous? Actually who are you not to be? You are a child of God. Your playing small doesn't serve the world. There's nothing enlightened about shrinking so that other people won't feel insecure around you. We are all meant to shine, as children do. As we let our own light shine, we unconsciously give other people permission to do the same. As we're liberated from our own fear, our presence automatically liberates others."

Nelson Mandela
(Quoting from Marianne Williamson's "A Return to Love: A Reflection on a Course in Miracles").

Heather Wright

Quick Recall Guide

Use this as a quick reference for your development ...

Page 34	Quick recall 1
Page 59	Quick recall 2
Page 84	Quick recall 3
Page 112	Quick recall 4
Page 138	Quick recall 5
Page 164	Quick recall 6
Page 183	Quick recall 7
Page 206	Quick recall 8
Page 226	Quick recall 9
Page 246	Quick recall 10

Acknowledgements for "Breaking The Mirror"

Page 1   T.E. Lawrence "*Seven Pillars of Wisdom*", Wordsworth Editions Ltd, New Ed Editions, published 1997

Page 17   Mark Twain

Page 21   Charles Swindoll "*Growing Strong in the Seasons of Life*", Insight for Living and also thanks to Joanna Bowles from Insight for Living

Page 35   James Baldwin

Page 51   Helen Keller

Page 60   George Bernard Shaw

Page 67   W. Clement Stone

Page 85   William Makepeace Thackeray "*Vanity Fair*", Penguin Books Ltd, New Ed Edition (1994)

Page 97   Arthur Ashe – from an interview

Page 109   Sir Paul McCartney from an interview

Page 113   Mihaly Csikszentmihalyi

Page 130   Sir Roger Bannister *"The First Four Minutes"*, Sutton Publishing, Limited Edition, 2004

Page 131   Vasiliy Alekseyev

Page 139   Tiger Woods

Page 152   *"The Lion King"* (1994), Walt Disney Pictures

Page 165   Shakti Gawain

Page 175   Lao Tsu

Page 184   *A Philosophy of Life* – Adapted from *"A Complete Treasury of Stories for Public Speakers."*

Page 195   Savage Garden *"Affirmation"*, Columbia Records, 2000

Page 207   John F. Kennedy

Page 208   Muhammad Ali

Page 209   Tommy Steele

Page 227   Johann Wolfgang Van Goethe

Page 233   Joyce Grenfell

Page 236   Spandau Ballet – "*Gold*" Chrysalis Records, 1983

Page 241   Monique Peterson "*The Little Big Book of Disney*", Disney Press, US, 1992

Page 249   Marianne Williamson "*s*", Harper Collins, New Ed Edition, 1996

Printed in the United States
94541LV00003B/208/A